PSYCHOLOGICAL INTERVENTIONS FOR CHILDREN WITH SENSORY DYSREGULATION

The Guilford Child and Adolescent Practitioner Series

Editors: John Piacentini *and* John T. Walkup

This series offers effective, innovative intervention strategies for today's child and adolescent practitioners. Focusing on persistent clinical challenges that cut across diagnoses and often come up in practice, books in the series present evidence-based tools for conceptualizing and addressing clients' individualized needs. These concise volumes provide what is missing from many evaluation and treatment manuals: the nuts-and-bolts techniques required for everyday clinical work. Each accessible guidebook includes a treasure trove of suggested interventions, complete with case examples, practical tips, sample dialogues, and practitioner-friendly resources, such as reproducible handouts and forms.

Teen Suicide Risk: A Practitioner Guide to Screening, Assessment, and Management
Cheryl A. King, Cynthia Ewell Foster, and Kelly M. Rogalski

Psychological Interventions for Children with Sensory Dysregulation
Ruth Goldfinger Golomb and Suzanne Mouton-Odum

Psychological Interventions for Children with Sensory Dysregulation

Ruth Goldfinger Golomb
Suzanne Mouton-Odum

Series Editors' Note by
John Piacentini and John T. Walkup

THE GUILFORD PRESS
New York   London

The authors have checked with sources believed to be reliable in their efforts to provide
information that is complete and generally in accord with the standards of practice that are
accepted at the time of publication. However, in view of the possibility of human error or
changes in behavioral, mental health, or medical sciences, neither the authors, nor the editors
and publisher, nor any other party who has been involved in the preparation or publication
of this work warrants that the information contained herein is in every respect accurate or
complete, and they are not responsible for any errors or omissions or the results obtained from
the use of such information. Readers are encouraged to confirm the information contained in
this book with other sources.

Library of Congress Cataloging-in-Publication Data

Names: Golomb, Ruth Goldfinger, author. | Mouton-Odum, Suzanne, author.
Title: Psychological interventions for children with sensory dysregulation /
   Ruth Goldfinger Golomb, Suzanne Mouton-Odum.
Description: New York : The Guilford Press, [2016] | Series: The Guilford
   child and adolescent practitioner series | Includes bibliographical references and index.
Identifiers: LCCN 2016001915 | ISBN 9781462527021 (hardcover : acid-free paper)
Subjects: LCSH: Sensory disorders in children—Treatment.
Classification: LCC RJ496.S44 G65 2016 | DDC 618.92/8—dc23
LC record available at *http://lccn.loc.gov/2016001915*

About the Authors

Ruth Goldfinger Golomb, LCPC, is a clinician at the Behavior Therapy Center of Greater Washington in Silver Spring, Maryland, where she has worked with children and adults with anxiety and related disorders since the mid-1980s. She has led many workshops, seminars, and training programs and has written articles for journals and newsletters. A member of the Scientific Advisory Board of the Trichotillomania Learning Center, Ms. Golomb is coauthor of two books, including *A Parent Guide to Hair Pulling Disorder* (with Suzanne Mouton-Odum).

Suzanne Mouton-Odum, PhD, is Clinical Assistant Professor in the Department of Psychiatry and Behavioral Sciences at Baylor College of Medicine and a psychologist in private practice in Houston, Texas. She has extensive training in cognitive-behavioral treatment for children, adolescents, and adults with anxiety and related disorders. Dr. Mouton-Odum is a member of the Scientific Advisory Board of the Trichotillomania Learning Center and past president of both the Texas Psychological Foundation and the Houston Psychological Association. She has published numerous scientific journal articles, presents at national conferences, and is coauthor of two books for the general public.

Series Editors' Note

In The Guilford Child and Adolescent Practitioner Series, our goal is to provide practitioners with a library of relatively short, practical, theory-driven books focused on common clinical problems and key intervention techniques. The books in this series differ from existing treatment manuals in that they do not focus on specific disorders, such as obsessive–compulsive disorder (OCD), major depression, or attention-deficit/hyperactivity disorder (ADHD), but rather on clinical issues that cut across specific syndromes or fall between the so-called diagnostic "cracks." These clinical challenges—including the treatment of sleep and somatic problems, sensory intolerance, unwanted habits, and adolescent noncompliance, among others—are common in children and adolescents in therapy, and are rarely covered to any useful degree in disorder-oriented treatment manuals. Yet these problems can have a profound impact on overall impairment, and even very well-trained clinicians can be perplexed by these complications of treatment.

By offering clearly and coherently organized volumes that provide highly practical, step-by-step guidance, we hope to help busy practitioners select and implement the assessment and intervention strategies best suited to their needs. Each book emphasizes the functional understanding of the antecedent (e.g., triggers) and consequent factors that serve to elicit and maintain the presenting problem. This theoretical framework provides a clear conceptual link between the target problem and specific assessment and treatment techniques. Ample case examples are used to illustrate case conceptualization and treatment selection and implementation. The technical aspects of the intervention are explained through clinical illustrations, sample dialogue, and handouts, forms, and other practitioner-friendly material.

Each book in the series provides relevant information about the topic problem, offering a clear description of how the behavior begins and is maintained, and how the problem may manifest and change over development and across different settings and contexts. The theoretical model underlying the problem behavior and intervention strategies are presented along with existing research support for these strategies. Guidelines for recognizing and addressing challenges that may arise during treatment are also detailed. Finally, given the common occurrence of the target behaviors covered in this series with other clinical problems, strategies for integrating the selected treatment into a more comprehensive treatment plan are provided.

This book by Ruth Goldfinger Golomb and Suzanne Mouton-Odom provides a full course of treatment for sensory dysregulation, also referred to as sensory intolerance or sensory processing issues. Children with this problem experience sounds, sensations, and other sensory input as highly unpleasant or even intolerable. Sensory dysregulation is commonly seen in children with a range of psychiatric problems, including anxiety, OCD, ADHD, oppositional defiant disorder, and autism spectrum disorders, and is often overlooked or misdiagnosed, which can lead to negative treatment outcomes and frustration among therapists, families, and patients.

The authors, both of whom are experts in behavioral treatments in general and in treatments for body-focused, repetitive behaviors such as hair-pulling disorder, skin-picking disorder, and the tic disorders in particular, draw from a very specific knowledge base regarding bodily sensations and their link to repetitive behaviors, and provide effective strategies to uncouple the sensations from the impairing repetitive behavior. Their systematic framework for evaluating and incorporating sensory data into the diagnostic formulation and treatment plan provides clinicians with concrete, well-tested strategies to help patients and their families develop the necessary self-management skills to reduce distress and improve overall functioning and quality of life. This book has done a wonderful job laying out the domain of sensory regulation and dysregulation, how to assess the problem, and how to treat it. Although there are similarities in treating anxiety and sensory dysregulation, habituation to the stimulus is not the goal of sensory dysregulation treatment. In this respect, the authors show that exposure approaches used in the anxiety disorders do not work with these children. The treatment instead focuses on helping children learn to manage and reduce the discomfort of the sensory difficulty by uncoupling the aversive sensory experience from the anxiety, avoidance, and negative emotions and cognitions that leads too often to catastrophic reactions.

Highly detailed case material and sample treatment plans provide therapists with the hands-on clinical material that is rarely available in treatment manuals. If you need expert guidance to deal with complex presentations of vexing symptom patterns, you've found the right book. Both of us have worked with the authors and have found their treatment plans to be helpful in improving outcomes in our patients with sensory dysregulation problems. We trust this clinically rich book will be eminently useful to you and the children and adults with sensory dysregulation difficulties whom you care for.

JOHN PIACENTINI, PHD
JOHN T. WALKUP, MD

Preface

Have you ever had a child in your office whose symptoms do not respond to empirically validated treatment that "should" work? Have you ever treated a child who exhibits symptoms of one or more psychological disorders, but something does not quite fit? When a child presents for treatment with complicated or treatment-resistant symptoms, it is like putting together a puzzle without all of the pieces. In cases such as these, the therapist may experience frustration, may blame the client for the lack of progress, or may give up on the case altogether. Often the missing puzzle piece is what we call sensory dysregulation, or a failure of the sensory system to accurately evaluate incoming information, resulting in symptoms or behaviors that mimic or complicate other psychological disorders.

Mental health professionals are trained in many areas relevant to the human puzzle: personality assessment, intellectual evaluation, clinical diagnostics, behavioral analysis and intervention, and family dynamics, to name a few. These professionals generally have less background in understanding the sensory nervous system (which processes information gathered internally and externally, organizes this information, and responds appropriately to sensory stimuli) and its direct impact on functioning. If therapists don't ask the right questions, they may make diagnostic assumptions that are incorrect, leading to misguided, ineffective interventions.

How does the sensory system affect emotional or psychological functioning? All of us use our senses to understand the world around us; however, each one of us perceives our world a little differently. This is true whether it involves a favorite color, genre of music, or variety of cuisine. Preferences such as these can shape hobbies, relationships, and career choices. For example, a person who has a keen eye for detail might grow up to be an architect, artist, or interior designer. Similarly, someone who is attuned to subtle changes in pitch might eventually write a symphony or play music as a hobby. Conversely, negative or unpleasant sensory experiences can also shape development in profound ways. What about the person who cannot stand the look of clutter or the individual who is very uncomfortable with the feeling of sand under his or her feet? These people grow up being shaped by their unique sensory experiences as well. Sometimes, these sensory experiences affect every part of a person's life. In more extreme cases, unpleasant sensory experiences can cause an anxious or unusual response and can present in the therapy office as psychopathology or as a complicating factor to a presenting condition.

What is meant by "sensory dysregulation"? Imagine having the flu, feeling like the only way to experience relief is to lie down in a quiet, dark room. Now imagine having the flu while listening to rap music turned to the highest volume and trying to study calculus. Every nerve ending in your body is reacting to the cacophony and the assortment of unpleasant physical stimuli (fever, aches, sore throat, nausea, pounding sound, and exhaustion), which makes it very difficult to stay focused and learn complicated mathematical concepts. Now consider living in that body at all times, with no relief except to avoid being around people or certain stimuli that aggravate your nervous system. It becomes easy to understand how people who have difficulty processing and modulating sensory information can become avoidant, anxious, impatient, irritable, depressed, or what we call dysregulated. Often therapists miss this important piece of the puzzle, which leads to misdiagnosis, improper or ineffective treatment, or treatment that goes well in the short term but ultimately leads to relapse. This book is a clinically useful tool for identifying when sensory dysregulation is a part of the diagnosis and what to do therapeutically to assist clients who frequently experience their world in ways that are unpleasant, offensive, or downright intolerable.

This book contains case presentations that are derived from composites of clients we have treated. All client information has been disguised to protect the identities of the individuals.

Contents

CHAPTER 1

Sensory Regulation and Dysregulation

Camille was having another complete meltdown. The sky was getting dark and it looked like rain. She began to panic with the first sign of a potential storm, even though she had never experienced a truly dangerous storm in real life. She would hide in her room with all of the curtains closed with the covers pulled over her head, screaming and in a complete panic until the sky started to clear. When she was in second grade, her parents were assured by the pediatrician that Camille would outgrow this fear and advised to ignore it, but the bizarre behavior continued to escalate. In third grade Camille saw a psychologist for 1 year to treat her storm anxiety, but with little benefit despite repeated exposure to storms and the experience of bad weather. In fact, the repeated exposure to storms (having her watch the storm from the window, listening to recordings of storms, watching movies about storms) seemed to cause her fears to get worse and her avoidance and acting-out behavior to burgeon. Camille is now in fifth grade and her anxiety is much worse, affecting her ability to maintain friendships, causing her to miss school, and exhausting her parents. Her therapist referred her to a psychiatrist for a medication consult because she was not responding to exposure treatment as expected. She was placed on an antidepressant medication, a selective serotonin reuptake inhibitor (SSRI) with little benefit, and her reaction to storms continued despite therapy and medication. Over time, her therapist stopped seeing Camille, as she felt unable to help her. Camille felt like a failure and her parents felt helpless.

Almost every mental health professional has had experiences with patients where treatment was not as successful as expected. Sometimes these cases are referred to as treatment resistant. Therapists may use evidence-based therapeutic approaches and still have poor treatment outcomes. Why does this happen? Although there could be many reasons why treatment does not progress as expected, such as poor compliance, family discord, environmental stress, and comorbid conditions, one important aspect that might be overlooked is the phenomenon known as sensory dysregulation. Sensory dysregulation is an emotional or behavioral disturbance that occurs when your nervous system is not perceiving or processing internal or external sensory stimuli accurately. The nervous system dysfunction causes either intense discomfort or the seeking of comfort in atypical ways. In children, the avoidance of discomfort or inappropriate comfort seeking to increase a positive experience can look like either anxiety or another psychological disorder. When sensory dysregulation is not identified as the problem or as contributing to the problem, good treatment can get derailed. Assessing for and treating sensory dysregulation in children helps psychological treatment progress more effectively, and the rate of relapse is reduced. Before describing how sensory issues can impact a child's functioning, we will give a brief, simplified review of the nervous system and the different functions that are governed within this system.

OVERVIEW OF THE NERVOUS SYSTEM

The nervous system sends electrical signals to different areas of our bodies to coordinate voluntary and involuntary actions, such as walking (voluntary) and digestion (involuntary), based on information received both from within our body and from its interaction with the environment. The nervous system encompasses two main parts: the central nervous system and the peripheral nervous system. The central nervous system consists of the brain and the spinal cord (which evaluate incoming information and give directions based on it), while the peripheral nervous system is made up of bundles of nerves that receive information from the environment and communicate between the central nervous system and the rest of the body to achieve homeostasis (a relatively stable state of equilibrium). The nervous system is engaged almost constantly in two important homeostatic functions: arousal and calming. Arousal or activation in an individual is governed by the sympathetic nervous system and is responsible for reactions such as excitement, fear, and self-protection. Calming, relaxing, and vegetative functions such as digestion and falling asleep are governed by the parasympathetic nervous system. These two systems are also involved in how an individual regulates the body and maintains a sense of equilibrium or comfort in response to environmental stimuli. The nervous system regulates itself through three main processes: sensory, integration, and motor:

1. *Sensory.* The sensory function of the nervous system involves collecting information both internally and from the environment using the sensory receptors found in the eyes, ears, nose, mouth, and skin, as well as in the skeleton and the organs that monitor the body's internal and external conditions. This information is then passed on to the central nervous system for processing by the somatic and visceral sensory nerves.

2. *Integration.* Integration is the process by which the many sensory signals that exist at a given moment are passed into the central nervous system to be processed. These signals are evaluated, compared, used for decision making, discarded as unimportant, or committed to memory as deemed appropriate.

3. *Motor.* Once the sensory information has been evaluated, an action will be decided upon. The action required may involve smooth, cardiac, skeletal muscle, or glandular tissue depending on whether or not it is voluntary or involuntary. Appropriate actions depend entirely upon correct interpretation (sensory) and evaluation (integration) of the stimuli.

The nervous system is constantly gathering and analyzing information garnered from multiple senses simultaneously, which allows one to experience one's environment as a complex but coherent whole. This combining and interpreting of multiple pieces of sensory information simultaneously is referred to as multisensory integration (Stein, Huneycutt, & Meredith, 1988; Stein & Meredith, 1993) and informs the individual how best to respond to specific stimuli (Ayres, 1958, 1961). Every person has a unique interpretation of sensory stimuli, which is why one person may be thrilled by the experience of a roller coaster hurtling downward at 60 miles an hour, while another might be nauseous and/or extremely uncomfortable with either the motion of the roller coaster, the sensations of the loud noise, the wind hitting her face, or the intense visual overload provided by the experience. Either way, each person's nervous system has gathered and evaluated sensory information, and consequently has directed that individual to respond in a way that will maintain individual comfort (seeking the roller coaster or avoiding it).

SENSORY REGULATION, LEARNING, AND BEHAVIOR

Information processed by the nervous system is important for learning, memory, and behavior. For example, a person who is prone to feel chilled in 65 degrees would likely bring a sweater to go out for the day in the belief that it is a cool day, while another person might wear shorts and a T-shirt the same day believing that the same weather conditions constitute a warm day. The nervous system is a powerful generator of knowledge and memories that lead to subjective belief and action.

Misunderstanding sensory-based issues can derail treatment in a variety of ways. For example, the goal of therapy frequently focuses on identifying and changing irrational thoughts and beliefs. However, dysregulation of the sensory system can lead to beliefs and actions that are appropriate in the context of that individual, but can be highly inappropriate in relation to the surrounding world. It can be tricky in therapy when a child presents as having what seem to be irrational beliefs based on her sensory experiences because to her the beliefs are quite rational—for example, "I can't stand the sound of thunder because it hurts my ears." Many children cannot articulate their feelings clearly, so the details about their discomfort do not get verbalized to parents or clinicians. A therapist may interpret this response to storms by assuming the child is afraid based on the irrational belief that "storms are dangerous." The therapist would likely attempt to change the erroneous belief through cognitive challenging and cognitive restructuring. The child's belief, however, is accurate (the sound of thunder does feel terrible and may indeed hurt her ears). The therapist could help this child by giving her a full understanding of her own nervous system and by developing new, creative ways for her to comfort herself in stressful situations (loud storms). Expanding the therapeutic understanding of childhood behavior leads to self-awareness, an ability to gain a sense of control when feelings are overwhelming, and confidence in being able to manage challenging situations in the future.

SENSORY REGULATION

The sensory nervous system works with all of the far senses—sight, smell, touch, hearing, and taste—as well as the near senses, such as proprioceptive (body position), interoceptive (internal organs), and vestibular (movement). A well-functioning nervous system gathers all pertinent information accurately, integrates it effectively, then makes decisions that lead to homeostasis. Sensory perceptions determine likes and dislikes in every way imaginable: decorating a house in a style that is pleasing to the eye, wearing perfume that is pleasing to the nose, listening to music that is pleasing to the ear, and so on. Each of us may have a different idea about what is satisfying to us. Our unique nervous system guides each of us to create a personally gratifying environment that suits our sensibilities.

The nervous system also alerts one to situations that are perceived to be uncomfortable. A loud rock concert is tolerable for some people, while spicy foods are inedible for others. Avoiding certain foods or loud music are just a few examples of how the system learns what is comfortable and what is unpleasant or offensive for each of us, and we make decisions accordingly.

The sympathetic nervous system also serves a safety function through activation or arousal in response to perceived danger. For example, if you're driving on a highway at a steady pace when the surrounding cars are speeding, but the car in front of you comes to an abrupt stop, you would immediately hit the brakes, without any conscious thought. This motor reaction may also be accompanied by involuntary responses such as rapid heartbeat, tense muscles, increased blood flow to internal organs, or an adrenaline boost. The sympathetic nervous system prepares the individual for immediate action if needed, also referred to as the fight, flight, or freeze response. When sensory stimuli are inaccurately perceived by the nervous system, the sympathetic nervous system can get triggered, resulting in the fight, flight, or freeze response. The stimuli are then perceived to be dangerous, as the self-preservation response occurs.

Everything described until now explains, in a rather simplified way, how the nervous system operates when it is working normally. However, sometimes sensations are experienced in either an exaggerated way or as insignificant when compared to how others experience them. These incorrect signals are sent to the central nervous system, and the system may respond as if they are accurate, for example, hearing a balloon popping and experiencing it as if it were a rifle firing right next to your ear. Furthermore, when there is a breakdown in the integration of sensory information (unimportant information is not discarded or the system experiences a sensory overload), mistakes in action or reaction can also occur. Children with these actions or reactions can appear in the therapy office misdiagnosed with a variety of different disorders, which will be discussed in detail in Chapter 8.

There is limited research about how internal sensory experiences evoke external behaviors or symptoms, but what does exist indicates that sensory sensitivities can impact behavior and functioning. For example, people with Tourette syndrome report heightened interoceptive awareness and a hypersensitivity to external stimuli for all five of the far senses (Belluscio, Jin, Watters, Lee, & Hallett, 2011; Eddy, Rickards, Critchley, & Cavanna, 2013; Woods, Miltenberger, & Flach, 1996), and people with obsessive–compulsive disorder (OCD) report hypersensitivity and intolerance of external stimuli (Wu, Lewin, Murphy, & Storch, 2014). Taylor, Conelea, McKay, Crowe, and Abramowitz (2014) found that people with greater self-reported sensory intolerance had a higher lifetime incidence of tics and OCD than those without sensory intolerance. Miller and colleagues (Miller, Reisman, McIntosh, & Simon 2001; Miller, Robinson, & Moulton, 2004) found that poor sensory regulation is correlated with problems with attention and poor emotion regulation. Calkins, Fox, and Marshall (1996) and Fox, Henderson, Rubin, Calkins, and Schmidt (2001) reported that sensory reactivity in children was related to fearfulness. Finally, Hopkins and colleagues (2008) described how sensory dysregulation was significantly related to both internalizing and externalizing symptoms.

SENSORY DYSREGULATION

When sensory information collected by the nervous system is inaccurately read, processed, integrated, or evaluated it can lead to a disruption in homeostasis, mood, or behavior and result in reduced or impaired participation in activities of daily living (Miller, Nielsen, Schoen, & Brett-Green, 2009). There are three possible types of breakdown in the sensory system: sensory modulation difficulties, sensory discrimination problems, and sensory-based motor disorder. Sensory modulation difficulties—difficulty regulating responses to sensory data—are the type that will primarily be described in this book.

Within sensory modulation difficulties, three main subtypes have been identified:

1. Sensory overresponsive: responds too much, for too long, or to stimuli of weak intensity.
2. Sensory underresponsive: responds too little or needs extremely strong stimulation to become aware of the stimulus.
3. Sensory seeking/craving: responds with intense searching for more or stronger stimulation (Miller et al., 2009).

All of these phenomena involve difficulty regulating responses to sensory stimuli. The children discussed throughout this book demonstrate how these problems processing sensory information can lead to, mimic, or exacerbate anxiety and other psychological disorders, and how children who are dysregulated respond atypically to cognitive-behavioral therapy (CBT) treatment for anxiety.

> Eight-year-old Brad was about to sit down to eat dinner with his family. He took one look at his dinner plate and started to cry, became angry, and left the kitchen upset. His parents were perplexed. They enforced the family rule that if he did not return to the kitchen, he could not eat dinner. Brad went without dinner that night. At bedtime, Brad told his mother that green peas were touching white potatoes and he could not eat knowing that they had touched. His explanation was that it didn't look right. From that point on, Brad felt it necessary to examine the dinner plate before committing to eat dinner with the family. All of the food had to be separated so that the different colors did not come in contact with each other. He was not able to eat in restaurants or at his grandparents' house or go to dinner at friends' houses because he was too concerned that the dinner plate would not look right and he would not be able to eat. The thought of eating away from home would send Brad into an anxious state where he would cry, throw things, and refuse to leave the house.

Brad's nervous system was telling him that it is wrong when different-colored foods touch each other. It caused him such discomfort that he could not tolerate it, and he responded in a way that allowed him to ease his physical and emotional feelings. Unfortunately, Brad's reaction was also intense, as if his life depended on his food looking right. This example illustrates how faulty processing of sensory data can lead to irrational beliefs and emotional and/or behavioral dysregulation such as anxiety, avoidance, and dysfunctional behavior.

THE SENSES AND HOW THEY RELATE TO DYSREGULATION

The following section will provide a brief overview of three types of sensory dysregulation: overresponsive, underresponsive and sensory seeking. In Chapter 2 we explore these phenomena in more detail.

Touch

- *Overresponsive children* typically avoid touching objects or people, and avoid being touched by other people. They can have extreme reactions to getting dirty, to certain textures of clothing or food, and to unexpected touch. They may also avoid getting their hair brushed, having a bowel movement, brushing their teeth, and playing in sand.
- *Underresponsive children* have to experience heightened or intense touch to register the sensation. They may hit or push children, hug tightly, wear clothing or shoes that are very tight, or bang objects (such as computer keyboards while typing) and typically are not being bothered by cold or hot sensations.
- *Tactile seekers* may seek out tactile sensations that seem strange such as touching all kinds of objects, touching people constantly, tapping, rubbing objects or people, and seeking out stimulation in inappropriate amounts or unusual ways.

Sight

- *Overresponsive children* can quickly become overwhelmed when there is too much in their visual field (toys, words, people, or things). They may have poor eye contact, appear inattentive, or even cover their eyes, especially when the lights are bright. Other times they may be hypervigilant or fearful of additional stimuli being put into their environment.
- *Underresponsive children* may not notice messes or visual overcrowding and are not bothered by bright lights. They may dislike empty space or prefer clutter.
- *Visual seekers* will seek out lots of color or patterns, they may not be bothered by messes or even prefer them, and may be more comfortable with, seek, or create chaotic environments.

Sound

- *Overresponsive children* may cover their ears to close out sounds. They may become highly reactive to common sounds that others may not even notice, like someone chewing crunchy food such as a carrot, the sound of a vacuum cleaner, the ticking of a clock, or the engine of a loud car.

- *Auditory underresponsive children* may not hear certain sounds that bother others, may not react to auditory cues, and may not notice competing sounds that would irritate other people (e.g., the radio and television on at the same time).
- *Auditory seekers* may like very loud music or prefer to have several sources of audio input going at once.

Smell

- *Overresponsive children* may strongly object to odors that others may not notice, such as an air freshener, certain food cooking, or a ripe banana. Reactions may include screaming, vomiting, or avoidance.
- *Underresponsive children* will not notice unpleasant smells and never complain about things smelling bad.
- *Olfactory seekers* may seek out smells or investigate the world through smell. You may see these kids smelling things in their environment, including books, pens, their underarm, a friend's foot, something they found on the floor, or their finger after touching something that another child might deem unpleasant.

Taste

- *Overresponsive children* may be unwilling to eat food with certain textures or temperature and may spit out food, gag, vomit, or cry when presented with certain foods.
- *Underresponsive children* will eat virtually anything without complaint, including foods such as strongly flavored fish, spicy sauces, and bitter tastes such as lemon.
- *Taste seekers* may explore new things with their mouth or tongue. They may lick objects, put them in their mouth, or even swallow them despite their being offensive to others or even dangerous.

SENSORY DYSREGULATION VERSUS
SENSORY INTEGRATION DYSFUNCTION

The term "sensory integration dysfunction" was first used by an occupational therapist named Jean Ayres (1966b, 1972b) to identify and describe individuals with atypical responses to sensory stimulation and was later described in the book *The Out-of-Sync Child* by Carol Stock Kranowitz (2005). The clinical condition is now known as sensory processing disorder (SPD). While earlier studies examined the functioning of individual sensory processes separately, current research on this phenomenon focuses on multisensory integration, studying the interaction of two or more sensory modalities concurrently.

The concept of sensory dysregulation described in this book is identical to sensory dysfunction in terms of its mechanism, but sensory dysregulation also refers to the emotional and behavioral outcomes of a nervous system that is not functioning within the normal range. Sensory dysregulation is the result of a disturbance in the sensory system (including sensory integration dysfunction and/or SPD), but it goes on to encompass dysfunctional emotions and behaviors that are complex to both conceptualize and treat. This book is not intended to replace or to diminish the work being done within the occupational therapy realm; rather, it is an attempt to expand the understanding of the sensory system to mental health practitioners and explain how it governs far more than just a child's reactions to certain stimuli. This book describes how emotional and behavioral dysfunction can be the result of a glitch in the sensory system and how incorporating the evaluation of the sensory system into routine clinical conceptualization and treatment can help to enhance and improve outcomes in many complicated cases.

AUTISM AND
AUTISM SPECTRUM DISORDERS

This book intentionally leaves out autism and autism spectrum disorders (ASD) co-occurring with sensory dysregulation, not because this is not an important relationship, but because it is critical. All people with autism or ASD have sensory dysregulation issues, while a much smaller percentage of people with sensory dysregulation issues have autism or ASD. In order to successfully treat autism and ASD, one must be specifically trained. This book will not attempt to tackle this complicated and important treatment, not through oversight, but by design. The focus of this book will be to address sensory dysregulation when it occurs outside of autism and ASD and enters the realm of anxiety and other disorders of infancy and childhood.

> Johnny is a 5-year-old boy whose mother brought him in for evaluation after his kindergarten teacher expressed concerns about his unusual behavior. She reported that he is constantly touching, rubbing, smelling, and licking objects in the classroom, including his classmates. She stated, "It is as if Johnny does not know what an object is unless he has touched, smelled, and tasted it." His teacher seemed frustrated and annoyed when speaking to Johnny's mother, who was well aware of his strange habits. Since he was an infant, she remembered Johnny putting things in his mouth. She also reported that he has an unusually high tolerance for pain and will walk into the house with blood dripping down his leg from a cut that he does not even notice. Currently he is also unusually rough with his peers, not in an intentionally mean way, but in a roughhousing way that sometimes gets out of hand. Johnny is a talkative child who seems to want to do the right thing, but he continues to engage in behaviors that get him into trouble. Johnny shows remorse for his behavior but is unable to consistently correct his behavior. Johnny does not meet criteria for autism or an ASD.

Johnny is a good example of a child with a sensory-seeking nervous system, one who craves sensory input through smell, taste, and touch in a more excessive way than is usual. This is also evident in his high pain threshold, also an example of an underresponsive nervous system. Sensory dysregulation can cause not only obvious social difficulties, such as is the case of Johnny, but also more subtle and hard to identify interpersonal difficulties that may get misidentified. Over time, these interpersonal difficulties can develop into patterns of interpersonal conflict or avoidance, or problematic behaviors that start with sensory dysregulation problems but can become full-blown psychological disorders. The following is an example of how sensory dysregulation affects the relationships of a high school girl with a sensitive nervous system in a much more elusive way.

> Thirteen-year-old Sarah was having trouble with her friendships again. She had always had a small group of close friends who understood her quirky nature and were forgiving of her hot-and-cold reactions to seemingly benign situations. They thought of it as her being "Sensitive Sarah." At lunch one day, Sarah was sitting at a table, with her friend Alice's back to her as Alice talked with Amy. Alice and Amy were laughing and talking together for almost the entire lunch. Sarah felt certain that they were purposely excluding her and that they must have known how upset she was, yet neither one of them said anything to her about it later in the day. This upset and eventually infuriated Sarah. She came home and disappeared into her room. Sarah did not come out of her room for the rest of the night. The next day Sarah claimed she had a stomachache and refused to go to school. She began to avoid Alice, Amy, and other girls, without explaining her feelings. Her friends were confused and, after a while, stopped calling and texting her to get together. Sarah felt isolated and angry. She began to believe that her friends were purposely hurting her feelings and therefore not worth it. Sarah began to withdraw socially and tried to avoid school whenever possible, claiming that she felt sick.

Even by teen standards, Sarah's reaction to feeling left out seems extreme. Sarah was unable to interpret this typical social situation because she has difficulty integrating multiple stimuli: a loud environment, the intense smell of the food, the visual chaos in the cafeteria, and the subtle social cues. In combination, all of these stimuli contributed to Sarah's confusion about her friends' behavior and resulted in her experiencing intensely hurt feelings. Rather than asking her friends if she could join in on the conversation, Sarah became overwhelmed and shut down emotionally. Her faulty assumptions perpetuated her hurt feelings and sense of isolation.

Sarah was also unable to both calm herself down and to talk to her friends about her feelings.

Accurately decoding situations contributes to emotional stability and regulation. The decoding process is an intrinsic function of the sensory system. Faulty decoding led Sarah to misunderstand her friends' behavior. This misunderstanding caused her to assume that her friends must have purposely ignored her, known how she felt, and not done anything to make her feel better. In addition to a faulty read of her environment, which made her anxious and angry, Sarah lacked the skills to manage those overwhelming feelings. Her emotional response was intense and confusing, which made her want to avoid similar experiences and ultimately caused her to withdraw from engaging in other relationships. Sarah's response to her friends' lunchtime chat is a good example of how a normal event can become a catalyst for emotional dysregulation and problematic behavioral responses that can have long-lasting implications.

DEVELOPMENT AND DYSREGULATION

According to Ayers (1966a), human development is dependent on three important neurobiological precepts:

1. Development follows a predictable sequence.
2. Abnormal development may reflect the expression of more primitive behavior.
3. Maturation is dependent on interaction with the environment.

When there is a disturbance in the evaluation, processing, or integration of sensory information, as described throughout this book, these neurobiological precepts can be interrupted. Camille, the child who was bothered by the sound of storms, clearly demonstrated primitive behavior (hiding, screaming, crying) and an inability to mature in her reaction to the sensory stimuli associated with storms (continued resistance and avoidance of storms). Typical therapy did not provide relief for Camille or her family because the origin of her resistance was not identified or addressed.

THE MISSING PIECE OF THE PUZZLE

Problems with sensory regulation coupled with anxiety and problematic behavior create a perfect storm for confusion and disruption of the family, frustration in therapy, and potential treatment failure. Consequently, it is always a good idea to screen for the presence of sensory difficulties during the initial intake. If present, specific treatment for these issues can make a significant difference in the ultimate outcome of treatment. Understanding a child's nervous system helps shed light on what may be causing the problem, as in the case of Brad, who was not able to eat food with comingled colors. Not knowing about his sensory sensitivities, a therapist might treat him as if he had an eating disorder or OCD, while the true etiology of his symptoms is sensory in nature. Treating Brad with exposure therapy alone might cause him to feel overwhelmed, frustrated, and misunderstood, and would possibly result in treatment resistance and noncompliance with therapeutic recommendations.

A unique and creative treatment approach that combines treatment for anxiety (exposure), direct treatment for symptoms of an over- or underresponsive nervous system (sensory interventions and coping skills training), and counterconditioning techniques will be described in detail in this book. Brad's treatment might include the practice of gradually mixing colorful objects, introducing sensory soothing techniques during exposure to color mixing, and teaching calming thoughts and relaxation skills, all of which will be explained in detail in later chapters. You will see how Brad will become more flexible with eating, and how these therapeutic skills will build his confidence and help him better understand his nervous system. Ultimately, treatment will enable him to effectively manage his responses and provide him with tools to maintain emotional stability in the future. In addition, his family will benefit from therapy by becoming more understanding and taking a more compassionate and supportive approach with him, without accommodating his anxiety or negatively reacting to symptoms of sensory dysregulation.

This book describes sensory dysregulation and explains how mental health professionals treating children with anxiety and other disorders as well as sensory dysregulation can improve their diagnostic conceptualization and treatment of these hard-to-treat children. The book outlines how children with sensory issues may be misdiagnosed or improperly treated and illustrates how these issues can complicate the clinical picture. Numerous creative strategies are offered for successful management of the dysregulated nervous system. With early intervention, children can develop important lifelong skills that will lead to creative problem solving, better emotion regulation, reduced anxiety, increased functioning during stress, improved family relationships, more empathy toward others, and successful management of their nervous systems.

CHAPTER 2

The Senses

This chapter provides an overview and an explanation of the normal range of central nervous system functioning and discusses emotions and behaviors that can manifest when the nervous system is dysregulated. Once all the pieces of the puzzle are understood, assessment can be done and a comprehensive treatment plan can be formulated. The nervous system's primary function is survival of the individual. This includes warning the individual of potential dangers, quickly reacting to stimuli that might cause harm or pain, and alerting the individual to internal events that are of concern (e.g., hunger, thirst, or needing to eliminate waste). This chapter will describe in greater detail what happens when the processing of sensory information goes smoothly, as in normal development, and how incorrectly processed information can lead to dysregulation of the individual, emotional instability, and behavioral problems.

OVERVIEW OF THE SENSES

Individuals receive information from outside the body through the five senses and from inside the body through a network of neurons in the muscles, digestive tract, joints, organs, and respiratory system. This information is processed and decisions are made accordingly. Sometimes multiple sensory experiences happen at once. For example, at Thanksgiving dinner one might smell food cooking, see relatives and friends, hear the conversations that occur, feel the cold air from outside or the warmth of the fireplace, and taste the food once it is served. In addition, internal events will occur in response to these external stimuli—sensations of hunger or salivation in the mouth, a rapid heartbeat during the football game on TV, or a need to use the restroom after eating and drinking. During any given activity, a number of sensations are experienced at the same time. This merging of sensations or processing of multiple sensory experiences at once provides information to the individual about what is going on in the present and about what is to come in the future. Data are immediately analyzed in the brain to direct the individual toward appropriate responses.

Senses not only inform individuals about the safety of the environment, but also provide important information that leads to appropriate action. For example, upon seeing a thick snakelike shape that seems to be moving while on a walk in the woods, one might experience a fight, flight, or freeze response by stopping, experiencing increased heart rate, and retreating quickly, only to discover what was thought to be a snake was indeed a large twig. Withdrawing from or avoiding frightening stimuli is normal and appropriate; however, if an individual processes environmental data incorrectly, behaviors will seem inappropriate or unusual. For example, a child who experiences loud noises as painful might run screaming from a birthday party when a balloon pops unexpectedly or might avoid birthday parties altogether. Senses also provide information about stimuli that are pleasing. A child who discovers that after removing a hair from her head, rubbing the cool, wet bulb at the end of a hair across her face feels really soothing and relaxing might start pulling out her hair to achieve this sensation. Before long, the child has a bald spot, which clearly can confuse both her and her parents. When the sensory system is able to perceive, process, and analyze information properly, a person will engage in appropriate responses to stimuli and will behave in predictable ways. This next section outlines in detail the different senses and how they process environmental information.

THE FAR AND NEAR SENSES

The Far Senses

Senses that evaluate information coming from outside of the body are referred to as the far senses. These senses are the ones that are most familiar (hearing, seeing, tasting, smelling, and touching).

We are conscious of these senses and have some control over them. These senses are used to visually distinguish between people in a crowd in order to find a familiar face, block out annoying sounds such as the whir of a vacuum cleaner, or allow for typing on a keyboard without looking at it. As the brain matures, it processes information in a more refined manner, enabling the body to respond in ways that create or enhance a satisfying environment.

The Near Senses

The internal senses, which are less familiar to most people, are often referred to as the near senses. The near senses include the interoceptive, vestibular, and proprioceptive. These senses are not within our control and cannot be directly observed. This group of senses keeps the body in internal homeostasis.

The interoceptive sense is the system that regulates the internal organs and is essential for survival. It governs functions such as heart rate, hunger, thirst, digestion, elimination, body temperature, sleep, mood, and state of arousal. When the interoceptive sense does not function efficiently, children are unable to determine when they are hungry, tired, needing to eliminate, or aroused. The resulting behaviors can range from whining and irritability to extreme oppositionality and explosive anger.

The vestibular sense governs movement, the sense of gravity, and physical stability, and is regulated through the inner ear. It controls balance, motion, coordination, and an internal sense of quiet or discomfort. This sense is unifying in that it forms a basic relationship between the individual, gravity, and the physical world. When a child has a vestibular system that is not performing, she can be in a constant state of discomfort, feeling nauseous, off balance, or at risk of falling.

The proprioceptive sense gathers information about body position in space through neurons in the muscles, ligaments, and joints. The information is then processed to judge perception about where one is in a space so that interaction with the external environment can be adequately managed. Children who experience dysfunction of the proprioceptive sense might bump into things, fall out of bed, accidentally break things, get into others' personal space, and often appear awkward or clumsy.

INFORMATION MODULATION

The brain modulates all of these sensory messages by balancing the flow of information coming into and being processed by the central nervous system, so that only pertinent data are used. This modulation process has three main responsibilities:

1. To inhibit unnecessary responses,
2. To habituate the individual to sensations that are persistent or repetitive, and
3. To discriminate between sensory stimuli.

At any given moment, a multitude of messages are entering the brain through the senses. Sensory gating is the ability of the central nervous system to inhibit responses to sensory stimuli that are redundant or irrelevant. Inhibition helps the brain filter information so that the individual attends only to sensory stimuli that are meaningful and require action, thus filtering out nonessential data and preventing inappropriate responses. For example, when you are walking the nervous system perceives drastic shifts in balance that, if taken as important data, might cause you to grab hold of a stable object to maintain balance. The brain, however, inhibits this response once the skill of walking has been achieved because the brain no longer needs to assess where and how to take the next step. Research indicates that children with sensory processing difficulties do not exhibit the expected maturation process with regard to sensory gating (Davies, Chang, & Gavin, 2009; Davies & Gavin, 2007). As a result, these children have difficulty filtering out nonessential data, which causes a multitude of problems with attention and concentration because they cannot ascertain which stimuli to attend to and get distracted by other, less important stimuli. This distraction can lead to being unable to focus on the task at hand, being overwhelmed in noisy, chaotic environments, impulsivity, and being easily being pulled off task. Another manifestation is for a child to become overly focused on one task while completely ignoring all other competing stimuli (including some that may need attention, such as eating, sleeping, or eliminating waste), such that he appears to be zoned out or in a trance.

Habituation occurs when sensory stimuli have been assessed and determined to be nonessential, and are eventually ignored. Examples of stimuli that are commonly habituated to by the brain are wearing a long-sleeved sweater, feeling the sensation of movement while riding in the car, or hearing a clock ticking in the classroom. In each of these cases, the stimuli might be noticeable at first, but become less noticeable or even negligible over time. Children who have difficulty habituating to sensory stimuli are keenly aware of that long-sleeved sweater (and often cannot tolerate how it feels on their body), never stop feeling the car's movement (and may become carsick or learn to hate riding in the car), or become focused on the clock ticking instead of the teacher's lesson. McIntosh, Miller, Shyu, and Hagerman (1999) studied children with sensory overresponsiveness and found that these children exhibited a larger reaction than the control group to all stimuli (sensory over-reaction) and failed to habituate to recurring sensory stimulation. Similar findings have also been reported in animal models (Schneider et al., 2007). This is precisely the reason why traditional exposure therapy, while highly effective for anxiety disorders, is incomplete for treating children who have underlying sensory processing issues—because they often do not habituate to the unpleasant stimulus. In Chapters 5 and 6 we will discuss specific ways to augment exposure therapy to make it more tolerable and ultimately more effective for use with this population.

Discrimination is the ability to tell the difference among sensory stimuli, such as knowing what an object is by looking at it without touching or smelling it, or differentiating between the different tastes and textures of food. Discrimination also helps individuals to be successful at playing sports, catching a glass of milk before it spills, or having the agile response to swerve out of the way of a car moving quickly into one's lane. Children who have difficulties with sensory discrimination (referred to as sensory discrimination disorder) receive confusing, jumbled, and inaccurate information through the sensory system, causing them to behave in strange ways, and can make learning terribly difficult. Sensory discrimination problems may be present in all seven sensory systems.

When the central nervous system does not function smoothly due to problems with perception, organization, or modulation of incoming information, a person's experience is markedly disturbed, sometimes causing behavioral problems that can be misunderstood or misdiagnosed. A simple way of thinking about these complex processes is that children who present with underlying sensory issues tend to fall into one of these categories for each of the senses, overresponsive, underresponsive, or sensory seekers regardless of the underlying dysfunction in the sensory system.

THE OVERRESPONSIVE CHILD

Children with oversensitive nervous systems can be described as sensitive or sensory overresponsive. These children tend to be overly responsive to sensory stimuli; they may become easily over-whelmed, and they often experience the extremely uncomfortable fight, flight, or freeze reaction to common, everyday sensations. This increased arousal can be quite distressing and confusing to the child as it is not clear why these intense, uncomfortable feel-ings are present. In addition to having strong sensations and emo-tions, these children are not able to identify the cues that caused their discomfort. In other words, not only are they confused about why they feel terrible, but they are also not able to determine how to prevent it from happening again. Sensitive children can experi-ence feelings of panic, generalized anxiety, and worry, feel out of control, or become completely stuck, unable to tolerate their sen-sory experience and incapable of escaping a similar outcome in the future. Children will often behave in ways that are no longer age appropriate, as Camille did. Over-sensitive children may cry, rock, run away, throw things, tantrum, avoid, fret, or insist on being held for hours at a time to avoid or attempt to ameliorate certain sensory experiences.

THE UNDERRESPONSIVE CHILD

Children with undersensitive nervous systems may be under-responsive to sensory stimuli and therefore do not notice sensa-tions that other children are acutely aware of. The undersensitive nervous system needs additional stimulation, more than the average person would require, in order to register sensory experiences. These children may eat sardines for lunch, walk into a stinky bathroom and not notice the smell, have food smeared on their face and not notice the feeling of the food, go too long without going to the bathroom and may have accidents, or may not notice loud sounds as they occur.

THE SENSORY-SEEKING CHILD

Children who are sensory seekers may crave sensory input and be described as engaging in unusual behaviors. These children search for sensory experiences that most people typically avoid or see as unpleasant or inappropriate. These children may present as compulsive masturbators, as kids who chronically jump off high ledges or furniture, overeaters to the point of obesity, or loud talkers who stand very close to people and may constantly touch others. Coupled with a reduced ability to accurately read the environment or social cues, these children can have tremendous social problems and difficultly establishing and maintaining relationships.

The following sections describe over- and underresponsiveness as well as sensory seekers of both the far and near senses. It is important to note that each sense is unique and not predictive of the others. In other words, a child may be overly sensitive to smell and love hard touch. It is not accurate to assume that a child is either overly sensitive or undersensitive across the sensory system.

DYSREGULATION OF THE FAR SENSES

Auditory Sense

Children who are overresponsive to noise experience intense discomfort in response to sound due to a dysfunction in gating (the ability to inhibit responses to irrelevant or redundant stimuli). Two subtypes of auditory overresponsiveness have been identified: those who are flooded by sounds and those who are unable to filter out background sounds (Kisley & Cornwell, 2006). In the former, children may cover their ears, scream, or cry when they hear loud, unexpected sounds such as fireworks, a fire alarm, or a car honking. The latter group may hate common household sounds such as the toilet flushing, someone eating crunchy foods, or the whir of the vacuum cleaner. Reactions range from covering the ears to having tantrums. Children will report that they are frightened by the noise, but in reality it may be that the noise is painful or overwhelming to the ears and ultimately the nervous system triggers the fight, flight, or freeze response. As a result of classical conditioning, children learn to fear or possibly avoid these situations, leading to school refusal (if there is the potential for a fire alarm or a noisy cafeteria), disruption of the family dinner (resulting from yelling at family members who chew loudly or interfering with familial relationships), or avoidance of using public restrooms (due to loud toilets and hand dryers). This sensitivity is also referred to as misophonia, defined as "the hatred of sound."

Noise-underresponsive children also have difficulty with auditory sensations, but in a much different way. These children may not respond to verbal cues, may talk very loudly even when the environment is quiet, may be confused about the origin of sounds, or frequently say "What?," and they tend to love very loud music and/or chaotic environments. These children often are uncomfortable or misbehave in environments that are silent or require quiet behavior (e.g., church, movies, classrooms, and libraries).

Noise seekers love loud sounds, loud music, auditory chaos, and commotion. These children are typically not bothered by loud, crowded places and may, in fact, enjoy them.

Oral Sense

Overresponsiveness to taste often manifests in children as eating issues. Mild overresponsiveness to food translates as picky eating and is fairly common. Children with more pronounced oral sensitivity have extreme preferences for food and often have a significantly limited dietary repertoire. They may gag or vomit when eating foods with certain tastes (salty, sour, sweet, tangy, or spicy) or have difficulty sucking, chewing, or swallowing. It is possible to be sensitive to oral–tactile senses, causing an extreme reaction to food texture (e.g., mushy or gritty foods). Sometimes oral-reactive children are reluctant to brush their teeth because of the strong taste of toothpaste. Oral sensitivity can impact nutrition, growth, dental health, family dynamics, and social development.

Oral-underresponsive children often love intensely flavored foods, even if they cause tearing, coughing, or burning sensations, drool excessively, and may chew on pens, pencils, or clothing.

Oral seekers often engage in behaviors such as licking, tasting, or chewing inedible objects. The world is explored through the mouth with these children. Parents are typically concerned about oral-seeking behaviors for health-related reasons (e.g., germs or choking hazards).

Olfactory Sense

Children who are overresponsive to olfactory stimuli are bothered or nauseated by strong smells and typically avoid places such as horse stables, public restrooms, or even the school cafeteria. In addition, some children may notice subtle smells that are typically not noticed by others, such as the scent of clothes after they have been laundered or the smell of something that has been wrapped in plastic.

Olfactory underresponsiveness includes the inability to notice noxious odors. It is often difficult for children with this problem to distinguish between different smells. They may like to eat foods with strong odors such as sardines, which may be offensive to other children in the cafeteria. Teenagers with this form of dysfunction may not notice their own body odor or bad breath, can be reluctant to bathe or wear deodorant, and may be observed smelling their fingers after touching parts of their bodies. Social encounters can become quite challenging as a result of this hyposensitivity.

Olfactory seekers have a desire to repeatedly smell objects in the environment or smell body odor from underarms, feet, or underwear. They seek out unusual smells, oftentimes at the expense of their social functioning.

Visual Sense

Overresponsiveness to visual stimuli includes photophobic reactions to sunlight or bright lights, insisting that things be ordered or arranged in certain ways (e.g., all shoes lined up in the closet), and avoidance of eye contact. Behaviorally, these children may be easily distracted by visual stimuli, refuse to read books that have narrow margins and small fonts, prefer solid-colored clothing, and become overly aroused by brightly colored or visually busy rooms.

Visually underresponsive children can have difficulty controlling their eye movements and tracking objects, often mix up similar letters, such as "p" and "q," or "b" and "d," tend to focus on minute details of a picture while missing the whole, have difficulty identifying objects that are partially hidden, are poor drivers, and have trouble reading maps. Behaviorally, these children will lose their place frequently while reading, tend to be poor readers, have difficulty copying from a book or blackboard, have cluttered rooms, can be disorganized and messy, and like bright colors.

Visual seekers will create visual chaos by making messes, spreading Legos around the room, or wearing completely mismatched clothing. Their bedrooms may be cluttered and overstimulating to most people.

Tactile Sense

Children who are tactile-overresponsive avoid messy play, are reluctant to cuddle, dislike light touch or kisses, and cannot stand rough clothing, seams in socks, or sand on their feet. Parents often spend hours in the morning with their children trying to get them ready for school, resulting in tardiness at school, intense family conflict, and potential job disruption for parents (lateness for work and/or inability to complete job-related tasks due to family demands and dysfunction). Contact with water can also be quite challenging, making baths or showers all but impossible to tolerate, and seemingly enjoyable family activities such as going to the beach with gritty sand, cool water, and sunscreen on the skin is often out of the question. Furthermore, tactile sensitivities can disrupt the parent–child bond when children dislike being touched or cuddled. Sometimes parents misunderstand this physical reluctance and react negatively to their own child, resulting in hurt feelings for both parent and child.

On the other hand, tactile underresponsive children do not realize that their hands or faces are dirty, they touch, tap, or rub objects in their environment, they may bump, hit, or scratch themselves without noticing, and often touch or play with others roughly. In addition, tactile hyposensitive children may have a very high tolerance for pain, bleed openly without noticing, or seek out painful experiences. This can be frightening to peers and interfere with friendship development. These children receive a great deal of negative feedback or correction from parents, caregivers, and teachers, resulting in complicated feelings for the child, who may feel unloved, misunderstood, and socially isolated.

Tactile seekers tend to touch everything, even when told not to. These children inspect everything by touch, including people and things that might be dangerous, such as hot stoves. Tactile-seeking children love massages, hugs, heavy blankets, and roughhousing.

DYSREGULATION OF THE NEAR SENSES

Interoceptive Sense

Children who are overresponsive to the interoceptive sense have difficulty regulating their internal environment. They may dislike the feeling of a rapidly beating heart, overeat or drink too much liquid to avoid the sensations of hunger and thirst, spend lots of time in the restroom to avoid feeling the need to eliminate waste or avoid going to the bathroom because the feeling of elimination itself is uncomfortable or even painful.

By contrast, children who are underresponsive to interoception may not notice feelings of hunger or thirst, or may seek out (seekers) activities that elevate heart rate. They might not be able to sense being full or satiated and eat large quantities of food, leading to obesity. They may not notice the need to eliminate waste and therefore are slow to potty train or have frequent accidents. Sometimes these children will like the feeling of hunger and therefore skip meals to feel hungry.

Vestibular Sense

Children who are overresponsive to the vestibular sense will often avoid playgrounds and moving equipment and are fearful of heights. Furthermore, these children typically dislike being tipped upside down, are unusually afraid of falling, avoid walking on uneven surfaces, and dislike rapid, sudden, or rotating movements. Behaviorally, these children may not go to the playground during recess, think going to Disney World is a terrible vacation, and avoid birthday parties with inflatable bounce houses. By doing so, they set themselves apart from their peers. These children may appear to be cautious, frightened, or shy, when in reality, they are simply reacting to certain types of movement.

By contrast, the vestibular underresponsive child or the vestibular seeker craves movement experience, especially fast motion or spinning. These children never seem to sit still and are thrill seekers. They shake their legs while sitting, love being tossed in the air, never seem to get dizzy, and are full of excess energy. These children may also set themselves apart from their peers because other children may not be able to keep up with the constant activity level and demand for more action. These children may be perceived as brave, adventuresome, hyperactive, or risk takers.

Proprioceptive Sense

The proprioceptive overresponsive child has difficulty understanding where her body is in relation to other objects. These children often seem clumsy, bump into things, appear stiff, and are uncoordinated. They do not like other people to move or even to touch their body, have a rigid or tense posture, and dislike stretching their limbs. They may also fear that objects are closer than they appear. They may become startled and overreact by jumping or ducking when an object is nowhere near them. These children have a lot of difficulty playing sports that require an accurate understanding of spatial relations or that involve running or being hit or tackled.

Underresponsive children or proprioceptive seekers are constantly jumping, crashing into things, and stomping. They are the typical "bull in a china shop" children. They love to be squished and get bear hugs, don't know how hard to push when opening a door, misjudge the weight of an object, are known to accidently break objects, and frequently rip paper while erasing due to pressing too hard. Underresponsive children prefer tight clothing, love roughhousing, and may be aggressive with other children. These children prefer sports where there is physical contact like football, basketball, and lacrosse.

THE IMPORTANCE OF UNDERSTANDING SENSORY DYSREGULATION

Children can experience a wide variety of sensory reactivity. Overresponders tend to be described as sensitive children who may be very emotional and avoid situations where repugnant sensory stimuli are present, as noted above. Underresponders are the children who either fail to recognize sensory input or seek out more sensory stimulation than other children. Interestingly, children can exhibit overresponsive reactions in some situations with certain stimuli and be underresponsive to stimuli in other circumstances. Therefore, careful analysis of a child's behavior is a key component to understanding the unique sensory experience of that child.

Every person has a nervous system, and each nervous system works a little differently. Before making assumptions about emotions and behavior, it is helpful to get some information about what sensory experiences may or may not be driving them. When the nervous system is over- or understimulated, irrational beliefs and dysregulation of emotions and behavior can occur. Over time, these thoughts, behaviors, and reactions (through reinforcement and conditioning) can develop into patterns and habits, which can appear in the therapy office as anxiety disorders, personality disorders, and other behavioral dysfunctions.

Children who have issues with sensory dysregulation are not always consistent in their presentation, which can further confuse parents and treatment providers. Symptoms may be more pronounced at some times and less noticeable at others. This might depend on environmental factors that either soothe or exacerbate the system. Careful analysis of the child and her internal experience, as well as environmental cues and triggers, can shed light on what factors contribute to or alleviate sensory difficulties. An important point to remember is that a child may exhibit characteristics of both over- and underresponsive to sensory stimuli in different areas of the far and near senses. The children described throughout this book have experienced sensory dysregulation to the point where it interferes with their daily functioning in a number of environments (e.g., school, home, and social). Furthermore, the sensory dysregulation issues affect their ability to establish and maintain loving, supportive, stable relationships with family members, caregivers, teachers, and peers.

The key to developing a comprehensive and effective treatment plan for any child in therapy is to fully understand the etiology, function, and context of the behavior itself. The next chapter outlines how to systematically evaluate and incorporate sensory data as a piece of the puzzle in the psychological treatment of children. Not every child with a psychological disorder has a dysregulated nervous system, but for those who do, it can profoundly impair functioning and, when missed, can complicate treatment outcomes and frustrate those involved in the treatment process.

CHAPTER 3

Assessing Sensory Dysregulation

To change dysfunctional behavior in children, therapists first must investigate the purpose and context of the behavior by developing a functional analysis at the onset of treatment. This functional analysis evaluates the specific behavior that is to be addressed, when the behavior happens most frequently, what cues (internal and external) are present that may trigger the behavior, and what factors may reinforce the behavior through reward (positive reinforcement) or removal of a negative stimulus (negative reinforcement). Of particular interest to this discussion are behaviors that are either a reaction to sensory experience or an attempt to somehow alter a sensory experience, resulting in a more pleasurable state for the individual. This chapter will outline how to incorporate the evaluation of sensory processing into the intake evaluation and functional analysis as a potential piece of the therapeutic puzzle.

EVALUATING FOR SENSORY DYSREGULATION IN THE CONTEXT OF THE INTAKE EVALUATION

When conducting a routine intake evaluation, many areas are investigated: family history of psychiatric disorders, the history of the presenting condition, developmental history, social history, academic history, and all aspects of the presenting concern. We recommend that some simple questions routinely be posed to alert the therapist to potential issues in the area of sensory dysregulation. First, it is important to ask parents about their child's early development. Often babies who were hard to settle, had difficulty sleeping and trouble establishing a routine, or were extremely fussy or colicky are the children who struggle from birth to settle their nervous systems and continue to be unusually sensitive to certain sensory stimuli. Conversely, babies who were not bothered by loud noises, bright lights, strong flavors or smells, hard tickling games, and roughhousing (being tossed in the air, spinning around, spending hours in a jumpy seat) are often the sensory-seeking children who require increased amounts of sensory input. Here is a typical conversation that might take place during an intake evaluation with a parent:

THERAPIST: So, Mrs. Smith, tell me how Sydney has responded in the past or currently responds to certain sensations like loud noises, scratchy tags, or socks. Was she sensitive to any particular sensations, as a child or even now?

MRS. SMITH: Well, now that you mention it, she was always very particular about her pants, she would only wear athletic shorts and would never wear blue jeans. I finally gave up trying to get her to wear long pants at all, even when it was very cold outside.

THERAPIST: Interesting, and did she mention what about long pants she did not like?

MRS. SMITH: Well, she would say that they hurt her legs, that she did not like the way they hugged her legs.

THERAPIST: How about now? Does she have any particular preferences for texture, clothing, food, or noise that you can think of?

MRS. SMITH: Now she loves very loud music, louder than I could stand, she says that it really calms her down. She also will only wear solid colors, preferably purple or green, and she will not wear white at all. Does she have OCD? It seems like she does because she will only wear certain colors, I think it is OCD and it drives me crazy.

THERAPIST: Let's look a little further into this. I have some additional questions I would like to ask about her sensory system before we draw any conclusions.

ASSESSMENT OF SENSORY PROCESSING

There are a host of measures available to evaluate sensory processing in children, but they are not typically used in the context of a psychological intake evaluation. As with the diagnosis of attention-deficit/hyperactivity disorder (ADHD), a combination of assessment methods is commonly used, including diagnostic interview, rating scales (examples include the Child Behavior Checklist [Achenbach, 1991], the Short Sensory Profile [Dunn, 1999b], the Infant/Toddler Sensory Profile [Dunn & Daniels, 2002], the Sensory Profile [Dunn, 1999a], and the Adolescent/Adult Sensory Profile [Dunn, 2002]), and behavioral observation. Occupational therapists can also assist with diagnosis when necessary.

Figure 3.1 presents a list of questions based on criteria from the sensory processing disorder checklist (Michelle Mitchell, *http://sensory-processing-disorder.com*, and Don Travis, *www.spdfoundation.net*) that we find helpful to screen for possible sensory dysregulation issues in children presenting for therapy. We recommend that these questions be used in some form during all intake evaluations as a quick screen for these issues. These questions are to be answered using a rating scale of 1–5, where 1 represents *no problem at all* and 5 indicates a *significant current issue*. "P" indicates that the problem was a previous issue but no longer causes difficulty for the child. Additionally, with older children, the questions can and should be asked directly to the child, as parents are not always aware of internal experiences that their child may have had along the way.

If further and more standardized information is needed, a referral to an occupational therapist may be warranted for a full battery of tests to evaluate the functioning of specific processes of the sensory nervous system.

Children who score above 4 on any subsection of this screening questionnaire often experience a variety of difficulties with

(*text continues on page 36*)

Does your child (Do you):

_____ Have unusual eating habits?
_____ Have unusual sleeping habits or sleep schedule?
_____ Have great difficulty with transitions (large life changes or small everyday occurrences)?
_____ Become engrossed in a single activity for long periods of time, tuning out everything else?
_____ Have difficulty with change in daily life or in the surrounding environment?

Oversensitivity to Sensory Stimulation

Does your child (Do you):

_____ Dislike getting splashed?
_____ Dislike the feel of sand at the beach?
_____ Avoid touching anything messy?
_____ Wash hands frequently or touch items through fabric?
_____ Hate to be barefoot, or hate to wear shoes or socks?
_____ Frequently get motion sickness?
_____ Avoid amusement park rides that drop, climb, spin, or go upside down?
_____ Prefer bland foods or dislike anything spicy?
_____ Become nauseated or gag from certain cooking, cleaning, perfume, or bodily odors?
_____ Become overstimulated when people come to the house or when in a crowd?
_____ React negatively to noises that other people are not bothered by (clocks, refrigerators, fans, people talking, blenders, vacuum cleaners, animals, etc.)?
_____ Overreact to loud noises, like sirens or thunder?
_____ Dislike patterns, bright colors, or stripes?
_____ Dislike messy environments or like things placed in a certain order?
_____ Dislike food that is touching together on the same plate?

Undersensitivity to Sensory Stimulation

Is your child (Are you):

_____ Unable to recognize stimuli that most would find alerting or strong?
_____ Unable to identify food that has gone bad by smell?
_____ Have difficulty being able to smell dangerous smells (smoke, noxious fumes, or something burning)?
_____ Unable to notice pain as others do?
_____ Lethargic?
_____ Unable to notice when hands or face are dirty?

FIGURE 3.1. Sensory processing disorder checklist. Based on the checklists by Michelle Mitchell, *http://sensory-processing-disorder.com*, and Don Travis, *www.spdfoundation.net*.

_____ Late in potty training (unable to identify an urge to go)?
_____ Slow or unable to catch self when falling or protect self from getting hurt; lacks reflexes?
_____ Unable to wake up in the morning, even with an alarm clock?

Sensory Seeking

Does your child (Do you):

_____ Love being touched, has to touch everything?
_____ Fidget with anything within reach all the time?
_____ Often touch, twist, or suck on hair (her own or others')?
_____ Love fast and/or dangerous rides and sports?
_____ Often rock or sway body back and forth while seated or standing still?
_____ Frequently tip chair back on two legs?
_____ Constantly chew on things?
_____ Prefer foods with strong tastes and flavors?
_____ Bite nails, fingers, lips, inside of cheeks?
_____ Love to sleep under multiple sheets and heavy blankets?
_____ Seek out crashing or "squishing" activities (may jump on furniture or run into people)?
_____ Frequently smell unfamiliar objects?
_____ Frequently lick or taste objects in the environment that others would not put in the mouth?

Sensory Discrimination

Does your child (Do you):

_____ Have difficulty finding items in a cupboard, drawer, in the closet, or on a grocery shelf?
_____ Have difficulty recognizing/interpreting/following traffic signs?
_____ Get disoriented and/or lost easily in stores or other buildings?
_____ Have difficulty concentrating on or watching a movie/TV show when there is background noise or distractions?
_____ Have difficulty remembering what people say?
_____ Have difficulty following directions if given two or three at a time?
_____ Talk too loud or too soft?
_____ Have difficulty eating an ice-cream cone neatly?
_____ Bump into things frequently?
_____ Push too hard on objects, accidentally breaking them?
_____ Often reverse numbers or letters or process them backward?
_____ Have difficulty telling time on an analog clock?
_____ Have difficulty reading and understanding a map, bus schedule, or directions?
_____ Have difficulty organizing or grouping things by categories, similarities, and/or differences?
_____ Have difficulty reading text on a computer screen?
_____ Have difficulty lining up numbers correctly for math problems and/or balancing a checkbook?

FIGURE 3.1. _(continued)_

Sensory-Based Motor Abilities

Does/did your child (Do you):

_____ Have difficulty learning to ride a bike, roller skate, skateboard, etc.?
_____ Have trouble because he/she is clumsy, uncoordinated, or accident prone?
_____ Have difficulty walking on uneven surfaces?
_____ Have trouble with fine-motor tasks, such as buttoning, zipping, tying, playing games with small parts, closing ziplock bags, etc.?
_____ Confuse left and right sides?
_____ Prefer sedentary tasks, avoiding sports or physical activities?
_____ Often hum or talk to self while concentrating on a task?
_____ Have difficulty learning new motor tasks or completing motor tasks with several steps?
_____ Lose balance frequently, maybe even while standing still?

Internal Regulation

Does your child (Do you):

_____ Have difficulty falling asleep or getting on a sleep schedule?

Is your child (Are you):

_____ Over- or undersensitive to bowel and bladder sensations?
_____ Over- or undersensitive to hunger and thirst?

Are there any other experiences that are very bothersome to your child (you) that I did not ask about?

Are there any other experiences that are particularly pleasurable or soothing to your child (you) that I did not ask about?

FIGURE 3.1. (*continued*)

social and emotional regulation. Specific over- or under-responsive reactions aside, these children often:

- Dislike changes in plans or routines
- Are stubborn, defiant, or uncooperative
- Are emotional and sensitive, prone to crying
- Are unable to finish tasks and projects
- Have difficulty making decisions, even simple ones
- Are rigid, bossy, and controlling
- Prefer solitary activities over group participation
- Are impatient and/or impulsive
- Have difficulty understanding social cues and nonverbal language

- Have difficulty with authority
- Have difficulty accepting defeat or forgiving themselves
- Are frequently angry and easily frustrated
- Experience many fears
- Experience panic attacks
- Are extremely particular; can't let certain foods touch each other, have to wear certain clothes
- Hate surprises
- Avoid eye contact

Over time, when left untreated, sensory-based issues can develop into other problematic behaviors such as avoidance of certain environments, oppositional reactions, rigid behavior, or social dysfunction. Children who have significant difficulties with multiple areas of sensory processing (scores of 4 or 5 on numerous questions in several categories) may experience extreme discomfort throughout childhood and often become dysregulated in their behavior, emotions, and sensory experiences. These children can be functioning well one minute and erupt with rage, panic, and frustration the next, causing their behavior to appear inconsistent or erratic. Furthermore, their reactions appear to be completely out of the blue, unrelated to the current situation, and as a result are perplexing to those around the child. Thus, when sensory dysregulation is present, it not only poses a challenge for the individual, but also profoundly affects those caring for or interacting with the child.

UNDERSTANDING THE FUNCTION OF BEHAVIORS

For some children, sensory dysregulation may help to explain maladaptive behaviors because they can be seen as a reaction to or avoidance of unpleasant stimuli, or an attempt to heighten a pleasant sensory experience. In this way, these behaviors can be viewed as serving a function for the child or at the very least, as understandable. For example, children who have a reactive arousal

system dislike surprises and have a strong need for their environment and routine to be the same every day. These children know
that change elicits an extremely uncomfortable feeling, so they are
not just resistant to change, but are frightened of how it makes them
feel. Parents, teachers, and other caretakers may view extreme reactions or inflexibility as oppositional, controlling, or pathological.

Understanding the functional nature of a child's behavior can
help parents and caregivers to be more empathic and less frustrated
when the child is displaying seemingly irrational or highly reactive
behaviors. Furthermore, functional information guides the therapist to select treatment strategies that address the etiology of the
problem without creating additional stress for the child. Therapy
can then include interventions that will assist the child in finding
alternate ways to increase positive sensory experiences and reduce
negative or unpleasant ones.

Figure 3.2 can help to clarify some of these functional aspects
when conducting an intake evaluation and is a variation of the
A-B-C model commonly used in CBT approaches and based on the
work of B. F. Skinner. For homework, ask parents to fill out this
form each time their child engages in the behavior(s) that concern
them. Remind them to be very specific about sensory aspects of the
environment that may have contributed to the behavior, particularly those endorsed in the screening questionnaire. After a week
of behavioral monitoring, discuss situations that tend to trigger the
concerning behavior and ways that the behavior serves a potential
function or is somehow reinforced. Information gleaned from this
form will help identify sensory-based triggers and outcomes that
will help inform treatment.

PROVIDING A DIFFERENT PERSPECTIVE

Identifying sensory-processing problems and how they relate to
presenting concerns helps us to better explain problematic behaviors. Remember Camille, the fifth grader who was frightened by
thunderstorms and became school avoidant? She was overresponsive to auditory stimuli such as loud, unpredictable thunder, which
resulted in a panic response and extreme avoidance. Knowing that

Antecedents: What was the situations or environment when the behavior occurred? What happened just before the behavior occurred? (places, situations, who is present, internal sensory experiences, as well as external triggers such as noise level, temperature, smells, tactile information [clothing included]).

Behavior: What was the specific behavior that occurred?

Consequences: What happened after the the child engaged in the behavior? (include changes in the child's state of being, as well as reactions from those around the child).

Date	Antecedents	Behaviors	Consequences

FIGURE 3.2. ABCs of behavior.

Camille's arousal system is highly reactive helps us to see that her extreme reactions make sense. Traditional CBT interventions such as exposure therapy or flooding alone are ineffective with a child like Camille, as the treatment often results in more discomfort, more helpless panic, or treatment refusal. Camille and children like her would not habituate to painful auditory sensations with exposure, and therapy could be ineffective. Camille's avoidant behavior is an attempt to control her auditory discomfort by avoiding the unpredictable noise of storms and, to her, is the only possible solution to a seemingly insurmountable problem. An approach that includes slowly introducing a hierarchical and graded exposure to the sounds of storms with the use of earplugs and soothing sensory input would likely be a more successful approach. This type of approach is based on Jean Ayres's (1972a, 1972b) work and includes employing multisensory environments while using challenging, goal-directed activities that are designed to provide specific sensory input. In addition, teaching calming cognitive and behavioral strategies for coping would target the associated anxiety and maladaptive cognitions and assist in relaxation. Finally, making these exposures fun by creating a game out of the exposure helps disassociate the discomfort from anxiety (counterconditioning). Over time and with practice Camille would learn to tolerate these uncomfortable noises and would eventually not react to them with panic and avoidance.

Johnny's experience, although quite different, was disruptive nonetheless. He would explore and enjoy his environment by touching, smelling, and licking any and all objects in his surroundings. He is a sensory-seeking child who interacts with his environment by acquiring sensory input from multiple sources. This unusual behavior makes sense now that we understand that Johnny, who requires a high level of sensory stimulation, is simply attempting to increase his pleasant sensory experiences while learning about his environment. Unfortunately, this behavior is also extremely off-putting to other children and downright alarming to adults. Finding appropriate ways to increase pleasurable olfactory and oral stimulation, such as using scented lotion, strong-smelling and -tasting gum, and sugar-free mints, while practicing behavioral inhibition would help to satisfy his sensory needs, and thus would decrease his need to inappropriately explore his world.

SENSORY DYSREGULATION CAN MIMIC OTHER DISORDERS

Children with sensory processing difficulties can present as having actual DSM-5 disorders such as OCD, panic disorder, specific phobia, social phobia, generalized anxiety disorder, or oppositional defiant disorder (ODD). In addition, disorders such as Tourette syndrome and ADHD can co-occur or be exacerbated by sensory processing issues.

SENSORY DYSREGULATION CAN COMPLICATE CLINICAL PRESENTATION

In addition to mimicking psychiatric disorders, sensory dysregulation can complicate the clinical presentation, making treatment frustrating for both the family and the therapist. For example, remember Brad from Chapter 1 who did not like his food to touch on the plate? One possible scenario of this treatment course over time would be that he continued to become oppositional at meals when things did not look right on his plate. Inadvertently, his parents might have reinforced his behavior by allowing him to leave the table and eat in private where he could separate his food accordingly. By being accommodated through negative reinforcement, Brad's challenging behavior might generalize to other situations where he simply did not want to participate, for nonsensory reasons. He might develop a habit of oppositional or avoidant behavior because it is easier than being with his family. If being in a crowded school with overwhelming visual stimuli is difficult for him as well, he may have similar reactions to school attendance and, as a result, develop an avoidance of school or even oppositional behavior, which could end up in poor academic performance or even dropping out altogether. Avoidance of social, academic, and other important life experiences could lead to low levels of self-confidence or lead to a belief that he is not able to handle situations that other children learn to manage through experience. If Brad presented for treatment at age 17 with this cluster of symptoms, it would require thorough analysis of the development and function of different behaviors over time and a unique approach to helping this young man develop skills in several different areas.

In the next chapter we explore in detail how sensory dysregulation may present as other disorders. We also describe how sensory dysregulation may co-occur with other disorders and how this comorbidity can complicate a clinical picture.

CHAPTER 4

It's Complicated

Sensory Dysregulation
and Other Psychiatric Disorders

In this chapter we briefly describe traditional cognitive-behavioral therapy (CBT) for anxiety disorders and explain why this type of approach alone may not work effectively for children who have issues with sensory dysregulation. Furthermore, we explore a variety of psychiatric disorders and examine how sensory dysregulation can obscure a diagnosis and potentially derail treatment.

TRADITIONAL TECHNIQUES
USED TO TREAT ANXIETY

As mentioned in the previous chapter, conducting a thorough functional assessment of a child's behavior illuminates the underlying cause of the behavior and leads to effective avenues of treatment. The cornerstone of any anxiety disorder is experiential avoidance (i.e., the child avoids situations that trigger anxiety in order to avoid experiencing the anxiety itself). As a result, anxiety disorders are typically treated using some form of exposure to the feared stimulus (experiential approach). Exposure techniques are used both in the office and between sessions and require the individual to face the feared stimulus (sometimes in a graduated manner) and experience the resulting discomfort without performing any action to reduce or escape the anxiety. Experiencing the discomfort of anxiety while in the presence of the stimulus (without avoiding or escaping the anxiety) allows the patient over time, to experience a natural reduction in anxiety called habituation. This process is repeated daily or several times a day until the initial stimulus no longer elicits a sharp spike in anxiety and a person learns that the feared stimulus is not, in fact, dangerous.

Exposure techniques are very successful for treating a variety of anxiety disorders including specific phobias, social phobia, panic disorder, and OCD, to name a few. This form of intervention allows a person to successfully turn toward and eventually learn to tolerate the uncomfortable feared stimuli and resultant feelings that fuel maladaptive behaviors such as avoidance, compulsive behaviors, or eruptions of anger. Unfortunately, exposure therapies that focus exclusively on experiential approach do not work effectively with a child who has issues with sensory dysregulation, but they can be modified to increase compliance and ultimately improve treatment success.

Traditional exposure therapy is ineffective and can be counterproductive when sensory discomfort is the primary cause of experiential avoidance, rather than fear or anxiety. For children with sensory dysregulation, habituation to the sensory irritant through traditional exposure therapy does not occur. They cannot inhibit the sensory information, therefore they cannot ignore, tune out, or habituate to the sensory experiences. In other words, although a child may have repeated exposure to the unpleasant sound, texture, sight, smell, taste, movement, or internal experience, his sensory discomfort persists because it is neurological in nature. At other times, habituation may appear to occur, only to have the symptoms return within months. When this happens, therapists can become confused or frustrated.

The goal of treatment when addressing sensory-based psychological problems is to help the child learn to tolerate her sensory discomfort while simultaneously learning to self-soothe and cope. Although sensory experiences do not change with repeated exposure (i.e., the loud noise still may be painful to hear), when treated properly, the anxiety that occurs as a reaction to the sensory experience *does* habituate; therefore the experience will no longer be frightening, just unpleasant. During this type of treatment, techniques for managing and reducing discomfort are employed (which is contraindicated in traditional exposure therapy) so that sensory discomfort can be decoupled from anxiety, avoidance, and negative emotion, rendering the experience less emotionally charged. Some of these management techniques include:

- Assessing the physical environment for specific sensory triggers,
- Adding sensory-distracting activities,
- Increasing self-soothing behaviors,
- Making exposures time limited and including counterconditioning, and
- Teaching parents how to emotionally support their child during the exposure to reduce anxiety and discomfort.

The specific details of creating a comprehensive and successful treatment plan will be discussed in Chapter 5.

HOW SENSORY DYSREGULATION CAN MASQUERADE AS ANXIETY

Sensory dysregulation can look very much like an anxiety disorder and is often misdiagnosed by well-trained and well-intentioned therapists. The following is a description of various sensory-based issues that appear in the therapy office as different anxiety disorders.

Obsessive–Compulsive Disorder

OCD is marked by obsessions or intrusive thoughts that raise anxiety and, as a result, lead to the performance of certain behaviors or rituals to reduce this anxiety. Over time the rituals become more and more frequent and evolve into an anxiety management tool that is short-lived and ineffective. The first clue that a child may have something other than OCD is the lack of a clear obsession. The following is a typical exchange between a therapist and a child who has compulsions with no obsessions.

> THERAPIST: Carl, what do you imagine will happen if you do not line up your pencils exactly right?
>
> CARL: I don't think anything will happen.
>
> THERAPIST: Why do you think you spend so much time lining up your pencils?
>
> CARL: Because if I don't, I won't feel right.
>
> THERAPIST: What will happen if you don't feel right?
>
> CARL: Well, I can't do anything until I line up my pencils just right. I feel terrible and I just don't like the way it feels.

This example indicates that Carl does not have any intrusive thoughts or beliefs about what might happen if he does not perform this behavior. He knows that he feels very anxious if he does not complete the compulsive act of lining up his pencils, but it is not clear why he must engage in this ritual. Now see how further inquiry by the therapist sheds light on his experience:

> THERAPIST: Carl, it sounds like it feels really bad when the pencils are not lined up, is that right?
>
> CARL: Yes, I feel very nervous.
>
> THERAPIST: I wonder if this nervous feeling has anything to do with the way the pencils look to you when they are messy. Do you ever feel like when you look at things that just don't look right to you, you have to fix them?
>
> CARL: Yes, they look messed up and like they need to be in order. I have the same feeling when I look at other things, like in my room I like to make sure the papers on my desk are straight and the pillows are even. It just looks so weird to me when they are not straight. Sometimes I even straighten a picture on a wall if it is crooked, but I usually do this when no one is looking because I don't want anyone to think I am strange.

Further inquiry about Carl's internal sensory experience uncovers important information for the therapist. Now the therapist not only has a better understanding of what is underlying the behavior, but has also uncovered other behaviors that can be used as practice during therapy. It is clear that the sensory experience of seeing pencils lined up is soothing to Carl's nervous system, while messed-up pencils are agitating. Carl has learned over time that this behavior of straightening things in his environment settles him down. Unfortunately, this straightening behavior is disruptive to smooth transitions, interferes with his ability to accomplish tasks in a timely fashion, and can result in Carl having an emotional outburst if pencils or other items in his environment don't look just right.

There is a type of OCD commonly referred to as "just right" and may be a manifestation of "Tourettic" OCD. It is diagnosed when no clear obsessions are indicated (Mansueto & Keuler, 2005). No research has been done with this subgroup of OCD sufferers to ascertain whether they simply have sensory dysregulation or if there is, in fact, a true just right/Tourettic OCD without the sensory component. Regardless, it is important to query about sensory experiences with these children to rule out an underlying sensory dysfunction.

"Just right" feelings can result from a variety of different sensory dysfunctions in addition to visual ones, and multiple maladaptive behaviors can manifest as and mimic OCD as a result. Here is a list of behaviors that are commonly sensory based and get mistaken for OCD behaviors:

- Lining items up so that they look right (visual)
- Ordering or arranging items so that colors are grouped together (visual)
- Having to wear certain clothes due to how they look (e.g., color, solid, print, pattern) (visual)
- Items such as sheets, blankets, or towels must look a certain way in order to use them—can include lacking dirt (where the dirt is not due to contamination), folded a certain way, or in a specific place (visual)

- Avoiding places/things due to how they smell (olfactory)
- Having to wear certain clothes due to how they feel (i.e., itchy, scratchy, soft, too tight, too loose) (touch)
- Avoiding touching certain objects or hand washing in response to hands feeling dirty or sticky (not due to contamination) (tactile)
- Avoiding foods/drinks due to taste aversions (taste)
- Avoiding/needing certain auditory stimuli (hearing)
- Must repeat behaviors until they feel right, not due to superstitious beliefs (interoceptive)
- Avoiding going to the bathroom or having ritualized toilet behaviors (interoceptive)
- Compulsive eating behaviors (interoceptive)
- Compulsive jumping, spinning, or cartwheeling behaviors (vestibular)
- Compulsive avoidance of activities that involve jumping, spinning, or cartwheeling (vestibular)
- Obsessions with risk-taking behaviors (vestibular)
- Tapping, rubbing, evening up that is not due to superstitious beliefs (proprioceptive)

The key to diagnosing children with underlying sensory dysregulation issues rather than OCD is to identify whether or not there is an actual fear or, conversely, a negative sensory experience underlying the behavior. The following are two examples of children who were diagnosed as having OCD. In each of these cases there is a lack of an obsessional system present; however, each child exhibits an exaggerated or unusual response to sensory stimuli.

Tyler, a 9-year-old boy, was brought to therapy by his parents, who were told by a psychiatrist that he had OCD. Tyler hopped into the office on his right foot. He would only hop, rather than walk, from place to place. Instead of sitting down on the couch or chair, Tyler squatted on the floor, again with only one foot touching the floor. His parents were at wit's end with Tyler's strange obsession with hopping and balancing. The therapist asked Tyler about the hopping and balancing. He stated that he cannot stand the way it feels for both feet to touch the floor at the same time. Even worse is when his bottom is on a chair and his feet touch the floor, it is simply too much. He learned that by only allowing one foot to touch at a time, he could reduce this unpleasant feeling and be somewhat comfortable.

Lilly was a 6-year-old girl diagnosed with OCD by her pediatrician, who was concerned about her washing behaviors. She had a history of hand washing that had really increased when she started first grade. Lilly frequently asked to leave class to go to the bathroom to wash and was known to wash up to 40 times a day at home. Lilly's parents were extremely frustrated and had started punishing her for washing, and had removed the soap from bathrooms around the house to reduce the drying of her hands. Most recently, she started refusing to put her underwear back on after using the restroom because she felt as if urine may have gotten on her underwear. Her parents were shocked and did not know how to handle this difficult situation, especially at school. When asked about her washing, Lilly simply stated that she does not like the way her hands feel when she has touched something. She feels sticky or like there is a film on her hands, even if there is no sticky residue on her hands. During the diagnostic phase the therapist and Lilly touched objects in the therapist's office, such as silly putty, and she became focused on going to wash her hands. She stated that she was not concerned about dirt or germs, she just does not like the way her hands feel. When asked about using the restroom and changing her underwear, Lilly stated that she can't stand the way it feels when even a drop of urine gets onto her underwear. She denied that the feeling had to do with contamination or the urine itself, it just feels terribly uncomfortable when the cold wetness touches her body. In an attempt to reduce the chances of her getting urine in her underwear, she would wipe for minutes at a time, leading to sore and chapped skin.

Both of these examples highlight how sensory sensitivities can mistakenly be seen as OCD if not recognized, and how this error could impact the efficacy of treatment.

Specific Phobia

Specific phobias are common in children and include fears such as dogs, cats, loud sounds, public restrooms, newspapers, people, and certain experiences such as roller coasters, riding a bicycle, long car trips, and a host of other stimuli. Parents usually bring their child to therapy after they have displayed very anxious or avoidant behavior in response to these or other triggers or the anxiety/avoidance is so frequent as to cause a problem with the child's functioning. When frightening events have happened to the child involving a stimulus, a phobia may develop. When there is no memory of a conditioned response (i.e., the child never had a bad experience or witnessed another person having a bad experience in this situation), sensory inquiry is worth pursuing. The following is an example of a child describing what looks like a fear of dogs.

> THERAPIST: So, Mary, I understand that you do not like dogs at all, they really scare you.
>
> MARY: I do not want to even see a dog or go into someone's house that has a dog, I just do not like them.
>
> THERAPIST: What are you afraid of? Did a dog ever scare you or bite you?
>
> MARY: No, I just don't like them.
>
> THERAPIST: Can you tell me about a time when you were close to a dog?
>
> MARY: Yes, a few years ago I used to go to my neighbor's house and her dog was smelly. He would put his wet nose on me and lick my hand and leg. I hate it when they get their wet tongue on me. I can't stand the way they smell and lick you all the time. People say that they are soft and the licks are kisses, but I think that their hair is wiry, yucky to touch, and I hate to have their slobber on my hands. I just scream and run if I see one so I don't have to touch it and it won't touch me.

This is an example of a phobic-like reaction to a sensory-based concern. Simple exposure therapy might be harsh and confusing to the child and may not yield long-lasting results. Other common triggers that can elicit a response such as anxious avoidance or panic reactions include the following:

- Loud toilets flushing leading to avoidance of restrooms or to not flushing toilets (auditory)
- Loud hand driers resulting in avoidance of public restrooms (auditory)
- The noise of fireworks leading to avoidance of any type of celebration where they may be present (auditory)
- Balloons popping eliciting avoidance of birthday parties (auditory)
- Certain animals causing avoidance of going to houses, parks, or public places where these animals might be present (auditory, touch, smell)
- Places with strong odors, such a public restrooms, stables, porta-potties, or certain restaurants, leading to aversions to these places (smell)
- Doing dishes (can't stand to see/smell all of the food mixed together) (visual, olfactory)
- Amusement parks and rides (can be due to vestibular experiences, sounds, smells, visual stimulation, or some combination of these)
- Long car rides leading to avoidance of family vacations, visiting relatives or friends, or going anywhere that requires a car ride lasting more than 20 minutes (vestibular)
- Eating certain foods (taste, texture, smell)
- Clothing (socks, shoes, pants, belts, dresses, turtlenecks, high-waisted, tight, or patterned clothes) leading to refusal to wear certain clothes, even if it is incongruent with environmental demands (e.g., wearing athletic shorts to church or wearing shorts when there is snow on the ground) (visual, touch)

The main point to remember when evaluating a specific phobia is to ask about the etiology of the child's reaction. Is the reaction to the stimulus truly fear based, or is it conditioned as a result of an unpleasant sensory experience that occurs with that stimulus?

Jacob was referred to treatment by his pediatrician for a fear of hand dryers. He stopped traveling anywhere with his parents that would require a rest stop on the way. In addition, Jacob refused to go out to restaurants with his family because the restroom might have a hand dryer. When discussing his aversion to hand dryers, Jacob described the loud noise they made as being extremely uncomfortable, leading him to scream and run out of the restroom, retreat back to the car, and cry, refusing to finish his dinner. Jacob's mother was able convince him to accompany the family to a restaurant only if she would go with him into the restroom and guard the hand dryer so that it would not be used while he was in the bathroom.

It is always important to inquire about why a child may be having a reaction. All too often therapists assume that the nature of the reaction is fear, and this is not always the case. Again, this can be confusing because children do develop fears of feeling uncomfortable. To distinguish between fear of a negative outcome (i.e., "there are germs in the bathroom that might make me sick") versus fears of feeling uncomfortable (i.e., "I can't stand the noise of the loud flushing toilet, and the way my ears hurt scares me") requires careful questioning and a willingness to consider that something other than irrational beliefs may be underlying the fear. Both scenarios involve fear and avoidance, but one fear is sensory based and the other is based on an irrational belief.

Social Phobia

Social phobia is defined as a fear of negative evaluation from others in certain environments that leads to extreme anxiety and avoidance of these situations. Sometimes, however, fear of social environments is not entirely the result of concerns about negative evaluation. Remember Sarah from Chapter 1 who had difficulty in the cafeteria with overstimulation by sounds and smells? She misinterpreted social interactions, assuming a negative evaluation of her by her friends due to faulty sensory processing. Eventually Sarah began to avoid social relationships in general. Due to her current behavior, she could be misdiagnosed with social phobia, and she may eventually develop a bona fide social phobia. Understanding the sensory aspects of her behavior would greatly facilitate and guide her therapy and lead to greater self-awareness.

> Jill was a 15-year-old 10th grader who had been avoiding large, crowded places for years, but it was now becoming a problem, as she was being invited to concerts, amusement parks, and other venues that she wanted to visit with her friends. Instead of assuming that her concern was due to fear of negative evaluation or even a fear of not being able to get out, as in panic disorder, her therapist inquired into her concerns. Jill reported that she can't stand the feeling of people touching her in a crowd, the noise, the visual stimulation of so many people together, and the overall chaos of the event. As a result, the therapist took a different approach.

Panic Disorder

Panic disorder is diagnosed when a person has a sudden onset of panicky feelings with no apparent stimulus other than a fear of feeling panicky. Children can be diagnosed with panic disorder when they have sudden rushes of unexplained anxiety and cannot verbalize the nature of their fear. Watch how targeted questioning can help to differentiate sensory dysregulation issues from true panic.

> THERAPIST: Tell me, Anthony, about your fears and panicky feelings.
>
> ANTHONY: Well, it happens a lot, I just start to feel weird.
>
> THERAPIST: Tell me about your weird feelings, what does that feel like?
>
> ANTHONY: Sometimes my stomach just hurts, it feels crampy and that makes me feel weird.
>
> THERAPIST: OK. What happens to you when your stomach hurts.
>
> ANTHONY: Well, I get really upset. I can't stand up straight, so I walk bent over. I start to breathe really fast and my heart beats fast too. I just can't stand it when my stomach starts to get tight. My heart beating really fast scares me and bending over helps that too.

THERAPIST: That sounds really awful. Is there anything that makes you feel better when you are feeling like that?

ANTHONY: My mom or nana will come in and sit with me. They will tell me funny stories and get my mind off of my stomach.

THERAPIST: What happens after you calm down?

ANTHONY: Usually I go use the bathroom and feel a lot better.

THERAPIST: Do you always go the bathroom after you calm down?

ANTHONY: Pretty much, yeah.

THERAPIST: I wonder if that cramping feeling in your stomach is your body's signal to you that you need to go to the bathroom?

ANTHONY: Oh, yeah, you might be right. But my body must not like to go to the bathroom because it really, really hurts.

Sensory processes seem to be underlying this child's discomfort. He likely has some interoceptive difficulties that make it painful for him to experience needing to defecate. Instead of reading those signals as "I need to go to the bathroom," he might read them as "I have a stomachache and that is really scary to me." In addition, not knowing the meaning of this signal might cause him to defecate less frequently, leading to more discomfort. Rather than having a panic disorder, he has problems with accurately reading his internal cues and has learned to respond with fear and trepidation (fight, flight, or freeze).

Disgust

Disgust is an interesting and important topic when discussing the sensory system. Like sensory issues, disgust may weave itself through a wide range of diagnoses and is often misinterpreted as other things. There is some current research studying disgust and how it affects the diagnosis and treatment of different anxiety disorders (Meunier & Tolin, 2009; Olatunji, Tart, Ciesielski, McGrath, & Smits, 2011). "Disgust" is defined in *Webster's* dictionary as "a strong feeling of dislike for something that has a very unpleasant appearance, taste, smell, etc." By definition, disgust is sensory based. When children have issues with sensory dysregulation, this strong feeling of dislike may present as anxiety, oppositionality, avoidance, refusal, or anger. An important area where disgust is a primary focus of treatment is emetophobia (fear of vomit or vomiting). Many times children with this problem can be misdiagnosed as having an eating disorder (limiting food to avoid the possibility of vomiting), school refusal (fear of getting sick or seeing someone else vomit), social anxiety (fear of vomiting in public), or a specific phobia (fear of seeing vomit or someone vomiting). However, disgust is not limited to fear of vomit. Many children find certain activities to be disgusting, such as emptying the trash, cleaning the dishes, scrubbing the toilet (not due to contamination fears), cleaning up after a dog, or toileting, and their disgust may result in anxious, avoidant behavior. In addition to activities, some objects can be considered disgusting, including roaches, spiders, rats, mice, or other rodents, certain foods, trash, blood, urine, feces, objects with specific textures, genitals, and physical irregularities of any kind (skin eruptions, scabs, warts, etc.) that may result in phobic-like responses. Here is an example of what might be mistaken for oppositional behavior but really stems from feelings of disgust:

THERAPIST: Tell me about your unwillingness to do your chores, Elizabeth.

ELIZABETH: Actually I do most of my chores, I just don't like doing the dishes.

THERAPIST: Really, I am curious about that, why the dishes?

ELIZABETH: Because seeing all of the food mashed together and all of the disgusting water going down the sink makes me want to throw up. I literally almost gag when I see it.

THERAPIST: So seeing the way it looks in the sink is the problem?

ELIZABETH: Well, it's not just the way it looks. It's also how it smells, how it feels, the whole experience is totally disgusting. I will do just about any chore as long as I don't have to do the dishes!

Misophonia

Misophonia is defined as a hatred of sound causing a person to react with anger or extreme frustration and frequently involves disgust. The sound of a person chewing food is often a trigger for a person with misophonia and is perceived to be disgusting. Other sounds, such as crumpling of paper or tapping, can elicit this rage reaction and can be misunderstood as a variety of behavioral disorders. Misophonia is a dysregulation of the sensory system that results in extreme anger. Treatment of misophonia also involves graduated exposure with the addition of sensory soothing, coping, and counterconditioning.

Attention-Deficit/Hyperactivity Disorder

Children with ADHD often present with an inability to maintain attention, difficulty staying on task, inability to complete multi-step directions, problems completing and turning in homework assignments, impulsive actions, and forgetfulness, among other behaviors. Children who have problems with sensory discrimination, a form of sensory dysregulation, may present with some of these same issues. These children often have difficulty with:

- Finding items in a desk, bag, or pocket
- Locating items in cupboard, drawer, or closet or on a grocery shelf
- Recognizing/interpreting/following traffic signs
- Concentrating when there is background noise
- Speaking at a reasonable volume (vs. too loud or too soft)
- Judging how hard to push on objects, often breaking things
- Telling time on an analog clock
- Organizing things by categories
- Lining up numbers correctly
- Remembering what people are saying

Children who are underresponsive to sensations may also have difficulty with sensory-seeking behaviors. These children often appear hyperactive, exhibiting behaviors such as:

- Loving to touch and be touched
- Fidgeting and fiddling with things all the time
- Loving fast and/or dangerous rides and sports
- Seeking out fast, spinning, and/or upside-down carnival rides
- Rocking or swaying body back and forth while seated or standing still
- Tipping the chair back on two legs
- Smelling or licking items to identify them
- Chewing or sucking on things constantly, including pencils, clothes, and fingers

Although these children display behaviors that are consistent with ADHD, the underlying reason may be sensory based. ADHD and sensory processing issues have a high rate of comorbidity (Kranowitz, 2005). For that reason, it is important to assess attention, concentration, and the sensory system when evaluating a child with these presenting concerns.

Tourette Syndrome and Chronic Tic Disorders

Children with Tourette syndrome or chronic tic disorders present with a range of tic behaviors, including vocal tics (throat clearing, grunting, sniffing, or saying certain words or syllables) and motor tics (facial grimaces, eye blinking, arm movements, or many complicated motor movements). Since tic disorders are neurological disorders, we know that the child's nervous system is functioning differently than those of children without tics. These children often have issues with sensory dysregulation. In addition to difficulties with sensory discrimination and sensory-seeking behaviors, such as occur with ADHD, these children may exhibit compulsive behaviors and are often diagnosed with OCD in addition to the chronic tic disorder. Sometimes sensory stimuli are experienced as a cue (premonitory sensation) and can elicit a tic or tic-like response. When treating children with tic disorders, it is very important to do a comprehensive evaluation of the sensory system, understanding how a child perceives different stimuli and how these perceptions impact his behaviors and emotions. With these children, it is always helpful to include multiple sensory interventions and self-soothing tools, in addition to the behavioral protocol for treating tics. These tools not only contribute to positive self-care but may also minimize certain tic behaviors.

BODY-FOCUSED REPETITIVE BEHAVIORS

Body-focused repetitive behaviors (BFRBs) include compulsive hair pulling, skin excoriation, skin picking, nail biting, nail picking, cuticle biting/picking, biting the inside of the cheek, and lip biting. For many children with BFRBs, sensory dysregulation is the cornerstone of the problematic behavior. Children who pull and pick often do so to reduce an unwanted sensory experience or to increase a pleasurable one. Examples of sensory-based pulling and picking behaviors are as follows:

- Pulling hair that looks different (thin, thick, curly, dark, white, out of place)
- Pulling hair that feels different (coarse, frail, sharp)
- Pulling to look at or feel the hair or hair bulb that is cool and wet
- Pulling hair to rub the hair or hair bulb along the face or lips
- Pulling hair to nibble the hair or hair bulb or to eat the hair or hair bulb
- Pulling hair to smell the hair or hair bulb
- Pulling hair to hear the eyelid slap on the eyeball
- Picking the skin to eliminate a scab or blemish to change the way it looks
- Picking the nail to smooth out the rough edge
- Picking the skin to eliminate a scab or blemish to change the way it feels (e.g., to make it smooth)
- Picking skin to see the excoriate come out
- Picking skin to smell the excoriate
- Picking skin to eat the scab or excoriate

- Picking skin to reduce the feeling of a bump, hangnail, or loose skin on the lip or cheek
- Biting the inside of the cheek to remove a bump
- Biting the lip to remove rough or dead skin
- Picking the skin around the finger- or toenail to remove loose or dead skin

Pulling and picking behaviors are also described by sufferers as meeting a deeper neurological need. People describe BFRBs as relaxing, calming, a tension-reducing behavior, or even stimulating and energizing. For many people with a BFRB, the entire reason for the behavior can be overlooked if this important sensory piece of the puzzle is neglected in therapy, resulting in incomplete treatment or treatment failure.

Caitlin is a 12-year-old girl who started pulling a few months ago. She pulled all of her eyelashes and eyebrows out and her parents were shocked. They immediately brought her to therapy to find out what was wrong with her and how to get her to stop this disfiguring behavior. When doing the functional analysis, her therapist learned that Caitlin started pulling her pubic hair as it initially grew in because it was coarser than her other hair, it felt different. At first she was intrigued by the dark, thick hair, then she came to believe that it "must not belong" because it had such a different texture. After a few weeks of pulling her pubic hair, she started to pull the eyelashes that felt coarser or thicker as well. Over time, she realized that the smooth skin on her brow and eyelid felt nice and she pulled any hair out to achieve the smooth feeling. Now, when hair starts to grow in, she immediately pulls it because it feels sharp and pokey to her fingers.

Caitlin is a typical example of a child with trichotillomania. Most children with trichotillomania or other body-focused repetitive behaviors pull or pick to reduce or achieve some sensory experience. When treating children with BFRBs, it is critical to evaluate the sensory system as it pertains to pulling and picking in order to develop a comprehensive treatment plan.

OPPOSITIONAL DEFIANT DISORDER

Oppositional defiant disorder (ODD) is characterized by a pattern of irritable mood, behavioral outbursts, and argumentative and defiant behaviors. Many children diagnosed with ODD also experience sensory dysregulation. In fact, many of their unpleasant, uncomfortable sensory experiences result in this pattern of ODD behaviors. Some examples of oppositional behaviors that also can be sensory based are as follows:

- Child is rigid about change.
- Child is described as stubborn, uncooperative, or defiant.
- Child is highly reactive and cries easily.
- Child has difficulty making decisions.
- Child can be seen as bossy and controlling.
- Child frequently gets angry or has moments of rage.
- Child hates surprises.
- Child may avoid eye contact.
- Child has trouble relating to and socializing with peers.

A therapist must pay close attention to the child's sensory experiences when evaluating for ODD. It is especially important to assess whether the behavior is truly defiant or results from avoidance of unpleasant sensory experiences. The following is an exchange with a child who was described by his parents and teachers as defiant.

THERAPIST: It sounds like you have been having some trouble at school, Michael. Can you tell me what kinds of things you get in trouble for?

MICHAEL: Well, I usually get in trouble for not doing what the teacher asks me to do, like sitting down in the morning and getting in line for lunch.

THERAPIST: Can you tell me why you don't sit down in your seat in the morning?

MICHAEL: Yes, the seat is really cold in the morning. It is so cold that I feel like it is freezing my butt and legs! Also, after lunch the seat in my other room is really scratchy, and I can't stand how it feels on my legs. I prefer to stand and not sit down.

THERAPIST: How about the lunch line, why don't you like to get in line?

MICHAEL: I hate it when the other kids touch me, it feels like I am being attacked when I stand in line, so I just stand out of line to avoid getting touched. If they want to send me to suspension for that, I guess I will just have to go.

Helping children understand how the nervous system functions and how to effectively manage internal and external sensory experiences is really important. When working with children, regardless of the diagnosis it helps to inquire about nervous system functioning and to properly address issues in this arena. Intervening at the sensory level could help change the trajectory of a child's life and most certainly can improve treatment effectiveness.

Treatment adjustments can be important and necessary when addressing two coexisting disorders that interact with one another, often rendering traditional treatment directed at a single disorder ineffective. In the treatment of Tourettic OCD, which blends features of both disorders, a treatment unique to the specific presentation is recommended (Mansueto & Keuler, 2005). When treating children with comorbid symptoms of sensory dysregulation and anxiety disorders, we propose an augmented treatment.

In the next chapter, we provide a step-by-step approach to treating sensory dysregulation in children. As stated earlier in this chapter, exposure therapy alone is incomplete as a treatment for children who also have issues with sensory dysregulation. The following equation indicates how treatment for SPD (Ayres, 1972b) can be combined with evidence-based CBT techniques to treat children with sensory dysregulation—a treatment that is described in detail in the next chapter.

Exposure + Sensory Intervention + Coping Skills + Counterconditioning = Tolerance for the Sensory Stimulus

The treatment goal is to teach these children how to manage their nervous system's responses to stimuli through a variety of interventions so that they can experience success in previously intolerable situations. Skill building and tolerance for discomfort helps children feel powerful and face difficult situations while learning about themselves and developing self-compassion at the same time.

CHAPTER 5

Treating Sensory Dysregulation
A Formula for Success

The previous chapters have shown how unidentified sensory dysregulation can be a major impediment to successfully treating children. This chapter explores our therapeutic approach to helping a child with sensory dysregulation. Often a therapist or family members will push a child with a dysregulated nervous system to participate in the very behavior he has had strong reactions to or has been avoiding. This often leads to anger and oppositional behavior and can affect the parent–child relationship. In fact, families often present with concerns about defiant behavior in their child for this very reason. Helping a child understand why he is having an aversive reaction is the first step toward change. Children feel validated and empowered once they understand how their unique nervous systems work and, more importantly, how their reactions and feelings can be successfully managed.

THERAPIST: Tell me about what happened in school, Sally.

SALLY: My friend Megan got me in trouble with the teacher.

THERAPIST: So what happened to upset Megan?

SALLY: Megan just started to cry and yell at me.

THERAPIST: What did Megan say to you when she was crying?

SALLY: She said, 'Stop it!'

THERAPIST: What was she referring to?

SALLY: Well, I was touching her. I like to touch her.

THERAPIST: Had she asked you to stop before she started to cry?

SALLY: Yes, but I like to touch her. Her skin is soft and feels good.

THERAPIST: I see. I think your body tells you that it feels good to touch certain things, is that right?

SALLY: That's right. I like to touch lots of things.

THERAPIST: I see. We want to find all sorts of interesting things for you to touch so that your body stays interested and happy. But it's also important to listen when people tell you that they don't want to be touched. How about you and I go on a hunt for lots of things that you might like to touch?

SALLY: That would fun.

THERAPIST: Then we will put some of those things in your pockets and your desk at school so that you touch those things when you need to touch something that feels good, and not upset your friends.

Simply providing information about a child's likes and dislikes directly addresses the issue and leads to solutions. In addition, it is important to normalize a child's experience without shaming her for engaging in either avoidance of or attraction to specific behaviors. These approach or avoidant behaviors feel good and serve a function, which is adaptive. The therapist's job is to find other, more socially appropriate, ways to get a need met, thus reinforcing a positive sensory experience.

As discussed in earlier chapters, it is important to conduct a functional analysis of the targeted behavior (identify all antecedents, behaviors, and consequences), to provide psychoeducation to the child and family about how problems with internal regulation can affect behavior and functioning, and to formulate a comprehensive treatment plan.

Ayres (1972) conceptualized treatment for sensory integration by providing a multisensory environment where challenging, goal-directed activities are designed to provide specific sensory input. More recently, Kim, Seitz, and Shams (2008), Ozdemir and

Akdemir (2009), and Frassinetti, Bolognini, and Làdavas (2002) demonstrated how using multisensory strategies improves behavior. Augmenting exposure therapy with additional sensory and cognitive elements helps dysregulated children successfully manage the nervous system's reactions. The formula that we recommend is:

Exposure + Sensory Intervention + Coping Skills +
Counterconditioning = Tolerance for the sensory stimulus

The remainder of this chapter focuses in detail on the individual pieces of the above formula, explaining how they can bolster a child's ability to tolerate the exposure work for successful treatment outcomes.

EXPOSURE

"Exposure" refers to the systematic introduction of uncomfortable stimuli (or something that approximates this experience) that, over time, will become less antagonistic. With regard to sensory experiences, exposure might involve tasting foods that are objectionable, going into a smelly bathroom, allowing the fire alarm to ring and not escape, and so forth. In therapy, psychoeducation about the importance and process of exposure work can set the stage for a child (and his parents) to get on board with this difficult work. If a child is opposed to the exposure, it is necessary to create a more modest, less objectionable experience first, to allow the child to have an opportunity to feel successful and build confidence. Exposures are typically ordered in hierarchical fashion from easiest to hardest, usually on a scale of 1–10, with 1's being the easiest and 10's being the most difficult exposures for the child. In therapy, this is referred to as an "exposure hierarchy."

How to Develop a Hierarchy

Once the functional analysis is complete, environmental factors, internal sensory experiences, and antecedents, behaviors, and consequences that trigger and sustain the presenting problem are identified (see Figure 3.2 in Chapter 3). Now it is time to break the approach to the uncomfortable situation down into manageable steps. In the case of Brad, who did not like his food touching on his plate, his therapist would initially discuss the benefits of being able to eat at school, go out to eat in restaurants, and eat at friends' and relatives' houses, essentially highlighting the benefits of behavior change. After reviewing the benefits of behavior change and gaining Brad's trust and interest in the process, the therapist would have Brad identify an action that would be somewhat challenging, but doable with little trouble (a 1 on the hierarchy). Then they might identify the absolute hardest thing he could imagine doing, something that would really make him uncomfortable (a 10 on the hierarchy). Next they would sort eight other actions that would comprise the 2–8 challenges on the hierarchy and write them down in order on a piece of paper. Here is an example of what his hierarchy might look like:

1. Place different-colored foods on separate plates to eat at the same meal.
2. Place a small amount of food of one color on a plate with different-colored food (greatly separated so that the two foods do not touch).
3. Place a larger amount of food on a plate with different-colored food.
4. Place two different-colored foods on a plate and have them touch.
5. Place three different-colored foods on a plate and have them touch.
6. Have a parent plate his food and then eat it as presented (with nothing touching).
7. Have a parent plate his food and then eat it as presented (with two foods touching).
8. Have a parent plate his food and then eat it as presented (with three foods touching).
9. Go to a friend or family member's house and eat their food as presented on the plate.
10. Go to a restaurant, order food, and eat what is presented without moving anything.

Brad would be instructed to practice each step or activity until it is mastered, and then he would move up the hierarchy to the next activity. When initially going through his hierarchy, Brad should be able to choose highly desirable foods for his exposure meals, for example, pizza and French fries to begin with while he is learning to tolerate seeing foods touch. This not only gives Brad a sense of control during this process, but also makes the exposure a treat instead of even more of a challenge. Once Brad has mastered the 10 exposures through doing repeated practice at each level, he should begin to experiment with different, more unusual foods. As with exposure-based interventions for anxiety disorders, exposure to the feared or uncomfortable stimulus is done in a systematic fashion, beginning with less provocative stimuli and increasing in difficulty as tolerance is built. The main difference is the addition of elements that make the experience more tolerable (rather than encouraging more and more discomfort). While this may seem inadvisable from a CBT standpoint (one would not encourage a client to resist or reduce anxiety during an exposure), it is necessary to provide these coping strategies for children who have problems with sensory regulation because habituation does not typically occur within the sensory system. The addition of coping skills and sensory soothing makes the exposure tolerable, thus reducing avoidance or the seeking of inappropriate sensory stimulation.

SENSORY INTERVENTION

With sensory dysregulation, children are prisoners of their own internal reactions. They are often confused and don't know how to make sense of their world, which is fraught with so many uncomfortable sensory experiences. Providing sensory experiences that either compete with or distract a child from discomfort can help to reduce the negative experience and make the exposure more tolerable. Sensory distraction (providing some pleasant sensory experience outside of the target behavior) or sensory substitution (creating a positive sensory experience that is similar to the target behavior) can provide the necessary sensory stimulation to allow the child to tolerate the uncomfortable therapeutic exposure or give her alternatives to the inappropriate target behavior. For example, Brad would be instructed to practice using sensory soothing while doing the exposures, such as holding a smooth stone in his hand or having some soothing music playing during the meal. These strategies could help Brad increase positive sensory input to help him cope with his negative sensory experience. It is important to experiment with a variety of different sensory interventions to see which ones work best, and in which environments.

Select Soothing Activities

Have the child take some time to experience each of her senses, paying close attention to what feels good. She should then explain what about the target behavior is unpleasant or particularly pleasing to guide discussion with the therapist.

> THERAPIST: What is it about socks that you don't like, Amy?
>
> AMY: Well, they just feel tight on my feet, and I hate the way the stitches at the end feel on my toes.
>
> THERAPIST: So, the socks feel tight and the stitches rub your toes?
>
> AMY: Yes, it is all I can feel until I take them off. My feet just feel so much better once I take off my socks. I can't even listen to the teacher when I am wearing socks.
>
> THERAPIST: I want you to look at these different socks that I asked your mom to buy during the week. She bought six different pairs that all feel different: some have no seams, some are very thin and lightweight, some are high while others are very short under your ankle. These are particularly soft and thin. What do you think of these when you touch them?
>
> AMY: I really like these, they are very soft and thin, and there is no seam.
>
> THERAPIST: I want to see if we could play a game where you put one sock on and leave it on for 1 minute.
>
> AMY: Do I have to put my shoe on?
>
> THERAPIST: No, not yet. Let's just see what it feels like to wear the sock alone for 1 minute, OK?

While the therapist in this example instructed the parent to make some specific purchases during the week, it is also helpful to have many objects with different sensory characteristics present in the office (maybe a basket filled with objects pleasing to the senses) so the child can explore different options. Have him touch and smell the objects while noticing which ones are pleasant and which ones are aversive. Having recordings handy on a computer or smartphone can also allow the child to explore the auditory sense. Many children already have some ideas about what items they like and don't like and will share these freely, but sometimes they discover new experiences they were not previously aware of liking or disliking. Each child should develop a list of possible sensations that are appealing or unappealing. Separate out the far senses of taste, smell, feel, sight, and sound. Have the child write down items he already knows of that are pleasing. Encourage him to explore each of the senses during the week and ask him to add to his list.

> Claire began to explore different sensory experiences and started to create a list. She went to a craft store and was reminded how much she liked to color. While at the store, she also felt some different-textured material and discovered that she liked the feel of satin and she also liked the feel of a feathery boa. Claire and her mother went to a home store and smelled different soaps, diffusers, and candles. Claire's mother bought a few soaps and a diffuser but was not comfortable with Claire having candles in her room. Mother and daughter then went to a kitchen store, and Claire discovered that she liked the texture of a bottle scrubber and a vegetable brush. Finally, Claire found some music that she really liked and created her own music collection so that she could listen to it any time she wanted.

Most importantly, sensory soothing should be utilized while a child is doing exposure work, both in the office and out. The therapist will assist the child in creating a plan for how to have these strategies available when she is in her world, outside of the therapy office. Claire should engage in an exposure (chosen from her hierarchy) in the therapy office first to practice using the soothing sensory items in conjunction with a challenging stimulus so she can see how they help her tolerate exposures and learn how important it is to have them available when presented with naturally occurring exposures.

COPING SKILLS

Children with sensory dysregulation can be taught techniques for developing coping skills—including relaxation, deep breathing, and cognitive restructuring—that can be used during difficult situations. As with sensory interventions, coping skills are taught prior to beginning exposure work because they are tools to be used with exposure. Once coping skills have been practiced and mastery has been achieved, exposure work can begin.

Relaxation

Relaxation training is an important tool to use when treating sensory dysregulation. Children who experience overresponsiveness become extremely uncomfortable very quickly. The discomfort is confusing, frightening, and anxiety provoking for many children because they do not understand why their bodies are reacting so strongly and, as a result, erroneously make the assumption that either something dangerous is in the environment or something is very wrong with them. In order to directly address the internal sensations, relaxation skills are introduced.

Relaxation training helps children slow down their reactions and calm their bodies. It is particularly useful with sensory-avoidant children as it helps them to achieve the needed sense of calm in situations that previously were intolerable. Sensory-seeking children also benefit from relaxation training because this gives them an internal sensory focus so they are not relying solely on external sources of sensory input.

The core concept of relaxation training for children is no different than for adults. The training begins with self-awareness and noticing the state of the body at any given time. Children should notice the difference in their body when they are feeling stressed or uncomfortable. Teaching progressive muscle relaxation and having a child practice daily to improve skills can prepare her for the rigors of the exposure process. As always when working with children, use simple language, encourage creativity from the child, and make the experience fun. For example, a therapist might ask a child to be as straight and rigid as possible, like an uncooked noodle. Then the child is instructed to cook in his seat. What happens to his arms and legs? How floppy can he become? The child has tightened his muscles while being rigid and relaxed them while pretending to be an overcooked noodle, thus illustrating the concepts of muscle relaxation for a younger child.

Breathing Retraining

When teaching breathing retraining skills to young children, a therapist may start with blowing bubbles. By showing a child how to take a big breath in, purse his lips, and blow slowly and steadily through the bubble ring, you can teach him to engage his diaphragm and support blowing out a long, slow breath. At home the child should pretend he is blowing bubbles and practice the deep breathing skill. He could also picture lots of bubbles as he blows. This method should be assigned for homework as well. The child should practice deep breathing each evening between therapy appointments.

Other ways to introduce deep breathing to a child include asking the child to count to five while breathing in and then holding the breath for three counts, then count to five while exhaling. Pretending to blow out candles on a cake is a creative way to engage very young children in breathing retraining. The child will need to take a slow, deep breath and then blow out all of the pretend candles.

No matter which strategy is used, the method for the deep breathing should be practiced in the therapist's office until the child feels comfortable using the skill. The therapist should also instruct her client about frequency and duration of practice between sessions. Remind the child she will not be able to use the technique effectively in the face of anxiety until the skill is well developed.

Cognitive Coping Statements

Many children experience maladaptive or scary thoughts during their unpleasant sensory experiences—thoughts these experiences have inappropriately taught them to have. It is important to discover the content of these cognitions so that they can be challenged. If the thoughts that occur with regard to sensory dysregulation are inaccurate, such as "I am going to die" or "This is the worst thing that could ever happen," the therapist and child should create more accurate statements that correct these thoughts, such as "I am not dying, I just feel uncomfortable right now," or "This is not my favorite feeling, but I can handle this." It may be helpful to refer to self-talk as best-friend talk. Children should be instructed to only say statements to themselves that they would say to their best friend in that situation. A child would probably not say "This is the worst thing that could ever happen to you" to her best friend, but rather something like "This is not so bad. You can do it."

Accurate statements that describe a child's nervous system can also be helpful, such as "I have a sensitive nervous system," "Most loud sounds are not dangerous, just loud," or "Certain things bother me more than they bother other people." Finally, children can use statements affirming that they have the ability to use their new tools and resources, such as "I can do my deep breathing," "I can relax my muscles," or "Smelling the perfume on my wrist will make this bathroom smell better so I can tolerate it for the next 5 minutes." Have older children keep a thought record where they monitor their irrational thoughts, as well as the more adaptive, challenge thoughts.

COUNTERCONDITIONING

Counterconditioning is a technique where an unpleasant experience is paired with a pleasant one, causing the unpleasant experience to become less noxious and therefore result in a more appropriate response. When working with children, using fun games during exposures helps to lessen the negative response to the exposure and increases motivation to approach behaviors that were previously refused or restricted. Games that are fun, exciting, and rewarding improve compliance and make therapy fun. Games might include having a fashion show to practice wearing new, not-so-comfortable clothes, pretending to have a spa where massages and facials are given to the child, or making the exposure progression a game, as in this example:

THERAPIST: Now we have an actual smoke detector and a recording of one that has the alarm blaring.

SCOTT: That's right, I have those at home.

THERAPIST: During the week each night I would like for you to play a game with your mom one night and your dad the next.

SCOTT: OK. What sort of game?

THERAPIST: First your mom will turn her back and you will have the actual smoke detector sound its alarm or play the recording that we found on the computer. Then your mom is to guess whether it was the real smoke detector or the recording. Then you turn your back and your mom will do the same for you, choosing one sound and having you guess whether it is real or the recording. The next night, do the same game with your dad.

SCOTT: OK.

THERAPIST: Remember, when it is your turn to guess, use your deep breathing techniques, and have the Silly Putty in your hand to help soothe you while you listen to the alarm.

SCOTT: Oh, yeah. I forgot about those.

THERAPIST: Also, you will earn points each time you play this game. The points will be earned for using the breathing techniques, using the Silly Putty, and listening to the sound without leaving the room.

SCOTT: That will be great!

Counterconditioning may increase a child's willingness to participate in certain exposures and can be an excellent technique for developing momentum during treatment. Other times, counterconditioning may not be necessary. At times a well-developed reward system is sufficient to enlist participation, if not enthusiasm, from young clients.

Developing a Reward System

Positive reinforcement helps children to engage in treatment more consistently and more readily. Immediate, tangible, desirable rewards are critical for some children to engage in behavior therapy both initially and throughout treatment. In addition to tangible rewards, verbal feedback from parents or caregivers reinforces behavior change as well—statements such as "Great job eating those peas and carrots," "Fantastic use of deep breathing," or "I am really proud of how you used the restroom at the restaurant." Over time, as you phase out the tangible rewards, the parents should continue with specific verbal rewards for the new behavior.

Reward systems help children to develop motivation for treatment, endure difficult steps during the therapy process, and navigate the process of behavior change. Reward systems don't always work, though. Most often when reward systems fail it is because they were poorly designed, too complicated, difficult to maintain, or inconsistently executed. Many therapists mention rewards but leave it up to the parent to develop a system. Because most parents don't know how to create an effective reward system, they create systems where expectations are too high, or rewards are too hard or take too long to earn or are not gratifying for the child, or the parent forgets to give the rewards. Therapists need to be involved in helping parents develop a reward system. Parents should be well informed, participate in the therapy sessions leading up to implementing the system at home, and feel able to modify and the manage the program at home. Small, medium, and large rewards should be discussed at the outset.

Here is an example of how a reward system can be introduced to a child during a therapy session:

THERAPIST: OK, now that we are clear on the exposure hierarchy, have identified some sensory soothing items, and have developed and practiced some coping skills, it is time to put it all together.

HELEN: OK, what do I do?

THERAPIST: This week, in addition to practicing your deep breathing and using your sensory soothing items, I want you to work on doing exposures that are 1's, 2's, and 3's on your hierarchy. Every time you do an exposure, you will earn points for the exposure and you will add them up at the end of the day. If you do a 1 four times, that earns four points, if you do a 2 six times, that earns 12 points. You get more points for doing higher exposures and for doing more repetitions of the exposures. Each day, I want you to try to earn more points for that day than you earned the day before. Make sense?

HELEN: Yes, it sounds like fun, but a lot of work too. What happens with all of the points?

THERAPIST: That is a good question. Do you want the points to help you earn something?

HELEN: That would be great. I have really wanted to get to have some friends spend the night. Maybe if I earn more points each day, I can have some friends spend the night on the weekend?

THERAPIST: Sounds like a good idea to me, let's ask your mom at the end of the session.

Parents should agree to all of the reward options and procedures. If the parent does not agree, then other options should be discussed until there is a consensus. Before the family starts working with the reward system, the parent needs to acquire the small rewards. Many families start this process before they have a supply of rewards in the home. This lack of preparation leads to frustration on the part of the child and is a good example of how reward systems quickly fall apart.

The reward system should be written out for the parent and child in a form that easy to follow and enables them to record progress. A chart is usually the best way to achieve this. The therapist should discuss where the chart will be kept (somewhere that is easily visible is usually most effective), as well as when the chart should be filled out (at a specified time each day). The therapist and child determine which behaviors to target for change each week. An example might look like this: Brad will eat a piece of pizza and a French fry that are on the same plate, practice deep breathing, keep his squishy ball in his hand during dinner, squeeze the ball on his lap, and review his coping statements with Mom before dinner. A daily reward might be a sticker on the chart for compliance and a weekly reward may be getting to do a fun activity on the weekend if five stickers were earned during the week. Brad and his parent(s) should agree to these parameters before leaving the office.

CONCLUSION

When sensory dysregulation is an issue affecting a child's behavior, treatment must include interventions that address the sensory system to make aversive stimuli more tolerable and improve the child's overall functioning. This chapter has outlined how to take information gathered in the functional analysis to construct an exposure hierarchy for the targeted stimuli or behavior with the addition of sensory interventions, coping strategies, and counterconditioning to enhance the impact of therapy. The next chapter describes interventions used for specific sensory sensitivities and provides an overview of how to incorporate them into the treatment formula discussed in this chapter.

CHAPTER 6

Specific Interventions for Over- and Underresponsive Children

When working with children who have issues with sensory regulation, it is important to make therapy as interesting and palatable as possible by adding pleasing sensory input to therapy, teaching important coping strategies, creating a fun, interactive structure for the child, and using rewards to encourage behavior change. This chapter explores the dysfunctions experienced by children with over- and undersensitivity to various forms of input from both the far and near senses, and introduces multiple treatment techniques for sensory dysregulation that put into practice the therapeutic equation Exposure + Sensory Intervention + Coping Skills + Counterconditioning = Tolerance for the sensory stimulus.

THE FAR SENSES

Olfactory

Children who have sensitivities with regard to awareness of smell can underexperience odors, which may lead to poor awareness of personal hygiene, or overexperience odors, which may cause avoidance of environments with strong odors such as public restrooms. Other times, they may seek olfactory information by constantly smelling objects or people. All of these behaviors can be regarded as unusual or strange, and children typically experience social repercussions.

Therapeutic techniques to address underresponsiveness to smell may include setting a schedule for regular showers, routine use of deodorant, and rules about laundering clothes after they have been worn once. While most children can smell their clothes and determine when they need to be laundered, children with sensory dysregulation have trouble determining when something smells or smells strong enough to warrant washing. Creating a schedule and rules that do not rely on their senses is a good technique to use with these underresponsive children. Rewards for sticking to the schedule are helpful to increase motivation for the child. Behavior charts that track compliance with tick marks or stickers so that a child can earn prizes can also be useful.

Overresponsive children have trouble entering spaces with strong smells and may benefit from using soothing sensory interventions, such as wearing essential oils (natural lavender, eucalyptus, or peppermint oil), pleasant-smelling lotions, perfume, or a pleasant-smelling aftershave on their wrists. If a child is resistant to these, try having her sniff an orange or other pleasant-smelling fruit while walking into the bathroom instead. Providing an alternate sensory experience that may mask or compete with foul odors can be an effective first step in encouraging the child to enter a space she was previously reluctant to enter. Rewards for entering smelly places can increase motivation.

Sensory seekers are children who are compelled to smell inappropriate objects or people. Strong, pleasant-smelling alternatives such as lemons or scented lotions should be made readily available for appropriate use. Alternatively, the child could chew strong-flavored gum or suck on very sour candy to satisfy this need. These strong smells and tastes serve as a sensory distraction as well as providing interesting sensory input, so sensory seekers will be less compelled to seek out odors inappropriately. Again, verbal praise and concrete rewards encourage behavior change.

> Ten-year-old Sam had been invited to go to the circus again. He had always wanted to see a circus, but avoided it due to his sensitivity to smell. Every year Sam would hear about the

acrobats, the clowns, and the fantastic costumes that the other kids saw and he would feel left out. Sam decided that he really wanted to go this year and talked to his therapist. Sam and his therapist practiced several interventions to help him tolerate unpleasant odors, such as entering the environment without avoidance (exposure) + chewing cinnamon gum (sensory distraction) + rubbing lavender oil under his nose (sensory input) + practicing relaxation skills (coping) while in the environment. These targeted interventions helped Sam to tolerate the smells of the circus, and he was truly able to enjoy himself. While the smells were still annoying to him, he was able to use his treatment plan successfully, which helped him feel proud and more confident for the future. His intrinsic reward was being able to go to the circus, something that he very much wanted to do.

Taste

Awareness of taste sensations includes underreaction to taste, resulting in being unable to identify foods that have gone bad or foods that are unappealing to other children. Overreaction to taste is often seen in children who are picky eaters or those who gag frequently. Sensory seekers are those who put objects in their mouths, regardless of whether or not this is appropriate to their environment.

For those who are underresponsive, it may be important to establish rules about what to taste and what not to taste, for example, teaching a child to take cues from others by noticing their behavior, facial reactions, and responses to food. A rule might be "Never put anything in your mouth that you are not sure is real food" or "Read the expiration date on foods before eating them."

Working with a child who is a picky eater can be a creative and fun experience for the child, parent, and therapist. Exposing a child to new foods in a novel way is a good start. Create a scene with food, such as cutting an apple and arranging the pieces to look like a face. This method may encourage the child to eat by using counterconditioning. Another example is to present "ants on a log" made out of celery stuffed with peanut butter, with raisins placed on top (counterconditioning). These creative food presentations engage the child's visual senses (sensory intervention) and lead to a less stressful and more positive atmosphere that will often encourage the child to explore foods that previously had been refused.

Children with an exaggerated gag response often have limited palates. To help children expand their food choices, start small. Create an exposure hierarchy that offers foods similar in texture to those foods that are well tolerated by the child. Encourage a very small piece or bite of a food to start, referred to as food exploring. Parents may offer small rewards for trying new foods using a predetermined reward system as described in Chapter 5. Parents often need help creating a manageable hierarchy of foods (exposure). A common mistake is for parents to insist that a child try a food that is dramatically different in texture, smell, and style from the foods that she currently eats. Pushing a child too fast, without sensory interventions and coping strategies, can cause the child to push back and create resistance to treatment altogether. Rewards for trying new and challenging foods help increase a child's motivation for progress.

Tactile

Tactile-underresponsive children may not respond to pain or not notice when something is hot, while overresponders may avoid others for fear of being touched, have extreme reactions to being dirty, or dislike brushing their teeth, wearing certain clothes, or having hair brushed. Sensory seekers will investigate tactile sensations in inappropriate ways (touching and/or rubbing all sorts of objects or people).

Outlining a set of rules for those children who are tactile underreactors may be very helpful—for example, "Assume the stove/iron/skillet is hot before touching" or "Do not play with knives/matches/scissors without a parent around to help."

Children who overreact to touch can have extreme reactions to feeling messy or dirty and to touching things that they perceive to be sticky or wet. Some children even find it difficult to eat a variety of foods due to the residue left on the lips, face, or hands while they are eating. These children often shy away from any experience that results in the feeling of excess particles on their skin. In cases such as this, the use of counterconditioning could be beneficial. For some children, creating a home spa experience could encourage exploration of a variety of textures on the face. The spa could start with a facial that includes a facial scrub or mud mask that requires time to dry on the skin. Once the facial is complete and skin is washed, apply cream to the cheeks and lip balm or makeup to the face. These experiences allow the child to feel the sensation of particles on the skin in a different and possibly rewarding context. If a spa is not of interest to the child, try creating a house of horrors by applying Halloween makeup and creating different frightening faces and creatures. The house of horrors might also include touching raw eggs or peeled grapes in a bowl (eyeballs) or touching overcooked, slimy noodles (guts) to make these experiences more fun and thus tolerable.

When children avoid others because they dislike being touched, a good technique is to create an obstacle course. This technique combines exposure with counterconditioning. The obstacle course should start at home using walls, furniture, family members, and stuffed animals as the obstacles. All family members should be well informed and aware that the goal of the obstacle course is to encourage touch and that the child will be bumping into and touching all items used in the course. Making a game out of this new behavior is designed to motivate the child to engage in and learn to tolerate touch while having fun at the same time.

For children who find brushing their teeth to be quite unpleasant, create a game of "beat the clock" and see if the child can keep brushing after the timer goes off. Set the timer for a very short time, 10 seconds to start, and extend the amount of time every few days. Another fun idea is to play a child's favorite song during tooth brushing, requiring that brushing continue until the song has ended.

Brushing hair can also be a challenge for children who are highly responsive to tactile input. Start by encouraging the child to brush her parent's hair. Experiment with different brushes and combs to see what feels best to the parent. Encourage the child to try the same items herself and see what feels best to her. Girls can play beauty parlor with parents or friends and wash/brush/style hair in a parlor atmosphere (counterconditioning).

Children who seek out tactile sensations benefit from creating their own sensory pouch (sensory intervention) full of interesting items to touch (soothing, exciting, or sensory stimulating). These items could include sandpaper, mini koosh balls, smooth stones, swatches of material that are interesting to touch, Silly Putty, a feather, pipe cleaners, or yarn). The child should be encouraged to keep this pouch in her pocket, backpack, or desk at school and to fidget with the contents when she needs some sensory input. The goal is to keep the nervous system regularly engaged with pleasant sensory experiences so she will be less likely to seek out other, less appropriate sensory experiences such as touching other children or objects.

Visual

Children with visual dysregulation can have difficulty looking at items that appear out of place or out of order, or may become overwhelmed with a lot of bright and/or colorful items in their visual field. Underresponsive children frequently have trouble making eye contact, are not bothered by bright lights, and can be extremely messy (enjoy having items scattered all over the floor). Overresponsive children react to visual stimuli with avoidance, acting out, or shutting down. When dealing with overly sensitive children, it is first important to create a relatively clutter-free atmosphere in the home. Developing a space that is soothing to the child can help him manage his nervous system on a daily basis. Next, introduce new items systematically, one at a time. Children can get used to more and more items over time, but it is important to begin with a fairly clutter-free environment. Next, the parent might create a game where an item is placed in a room where it does not belong (exposure). The goal is to keep the item in the wrong place for as long as possible. Another idea to help with exposure for visually sensitive children is to designate a "Waldo" item and play a game of Where's Waldo? in a crowded room (counterconditioning). Practice using *Where's Waldo?* books to introduce the idea of visual exposure to the child.

Younger children may appreciate incorporating their stuffed animal collection into therapy. Collect all of the stuffed animals in the house and have a huge family reunion, placing them all on the floor in a room (counterconditioning).The child may start by taking attendance. Parent and child may create some activities for the family reunion, such as nap time (putting all of the stuffed animals on the child's bed and having the child nap with her stuffed-animal family members) or teatime (providing tea and snacks for the family), both of which provide exposure. These are some examples of how to combine exposure with counterconditioning in order to encourage a child to interact with an environment that had previously been overwhelming and therefore avoided.

Systematic exposure and counterconditioning can be useful techniques for children who do not like the way things look when they are not straight (leading to shoes being lined up in the closet, pencils being arranged in a row in the desk, all colored clothes grouped together on a shelf or in the closet). Create an exposure hierarchy that slowly mixes things up, with a twist. Have the child make a game out of mismatching the shoe pairs or arranging the clothes by category (pants, shirts, etc.), not by color. Over time, the goal is to help the child become more and more comfortable with the look of things not being ordered.

When a child has trouble making eye contact, direct the child to notice something about people's eyes that is of interest. The therapist and the child might create a science experiment by having the child collect data regarding questions such as "What is the most common eye color of the people you speak with during the week?"; "How many people have eyebrows that touch in the middle?"; "How many people have long eyelashes?"; or "How many people wear glasses?" This exposure and counterconditioning technique encourages the child to look into the eyes of the people speaking to her while gathering data for the therapist. Here is an example of an older child who has difficulty with eye contact:

CHAZ: I have my first job interview in 2 weeks. I am hoping to work at our local grocery store after school and on weekends so that I can earn some spending money for college.

THERAPIST: That's exciting.

CHAZ: I am pretty nervous, though. I have heard stories about some interviews that didn't go well. What should I do to make sure the interview is successful?

THERAPIST: Well, you alone cannot guarantee that an interview is successful. You can, however, focus on your body language and present yourself as a friendly, interesting young man.

CHAZ: That's exactly what I want to do. How do I do that?

THERAPIST: Good question. Any thoughts about what conveys you to be an open, friendly person?

CHAZ: Well, my father has always told me that a firm handshake is important.

THERAPIST: That's a good start. What else?

CHAZ: Looking someone in the eye and smiling.

THERAPIST: I agree. How are those behaviors for you?

CHAZ: Not great. I know I have trouble looking people in the eye. I always have. It makes me really nervous, and I always look away. People think I am rude or uninterested. I'm not. I just can't stand to look into their eyes.

THERAPIST: That is a very good observation, Chaz. Are you interested in learning some techniques to help you maintain eye contact?

CHAZ: Yes.

THERAPIST: Sometimes when people are overwhelmed looking someone in the eye, they can focus on a different spot on the face. Let's try something. I would like for you to look at my nose while we talk. Can you try that?

CHAZ: Sure.

(*The therapist and Chaz talk about the upcoming interview for about 5 minutes, discussing how to talk about Chaz's classes, interests, and work history.*)

THERAPIST: OK, Chaz, we talked for a little while, and you continued to look at my nose while we talked. How was that?

CHAZ: Interesting. I did not feel as nervous. I was able to stick with it, which doesn't usually happen. Could you tell I was looking at your nose?

THERAPIST: No. What I saw was a young man interested in having a conversation and continuing to look at me the entire time. Well done.

Children who are underresponsive to visual stimuli can be drawn to messes, bright lights, mismatched clothing, and really wild-looking rooms. For those who really like the look of a mess, try allowing the mess, but have a rule that it must be contained. Parents can supply a large container where the child can put hundreds of Lego pieces, thousands of puzzle pieces, or a multitude of colored marbles. Allow the child to have the mess, but require that it be limited to the container. Rules about dress should be agreed upon to prevent negative feedback from peers, but parents must also understand that children should be allowed to express themselves through clothing. Sometimes it is more the parent anxiety that is the issue, not the child's actual behavior. Parent dynamics are discussed in detail in Chapter 7.

Auditory

Those who overrespond to noise often become frightened or overstimulated by loud or surprising sounds. Birthday parties with balloons, thunderstorms, loud flushing toilets, smoke detectors, loud concerts, and fire alarms can be intolerable for these children. Other times, subtle sounds can create a challenge, and they cannot filter out items such as a ticking clock, the humming of a computer, or another child clicking a pen in school. On the opposite end of the spectrum, children who are underresponsive to auditory stimuli prefer that the radio be on with the TV, like to listen to music at the highest volume setting, and can't stand to be in silence.

Overresponsive children (those who dislike loud noise) benefit greatly from learning coping skills such as relaxation training, which was discussed in the previous chapter. Instruct them to use those relaxation skills while working their way up the sound hierarchy. One way to create this exposure hierarchy is to have the child and her parent search the Internet for sounds. During the first exposure, the sound may be barely audible, with the volume increasing in subsequent exposures. Relaxation, deep breathing, and cognitive correction can all be used during exposure. Each time the child participates, she should receive some reinforcement or reward. As her confidence grows and her ability to tolerate sounds increases, she may enjoy making her own playlist of sounds. To increase tolerance for subtle noises, the child should practice listening to a clock ticking or a sound machine with white noise in the therapist's office. Employ strategies such as deep breathing, relaxation, counting the ticks, imagining that the white noise is the wind, or other creative sensory interventions that distract the child away from negative affect or physical states. Instead of trying to not hear the noise, have the child allow the noise to be there and, perhaps, be something else.

For those who are underresponsive to noise, once again the key is to employ rules, such as "Only one piece of equipment (TV, radio, stereo) on at time" or "Keep the volume on your iPod no higher than 7 in a public area of the house." The child can be allowed to listen at louder volumes (within reason) in the privacy of his room or while wearing earbuds or headphones to be respectful toward his family or friends. Self-monitoring of voice volume can help children recognize when their speech is too loud and self-correct. Listening to cues from others or purposely lowering the volume of their voice can help with awareness and behavior.

THE NEAR SENSES

Interoceptive

Children who overrespond to their internal states tend to dislike and have difficulty tolerating sensations such as a fast heartbeat, needing to use the restroom, actually using the restroom, and feeling hot or cold, or hungry or thirsty. On the other hand, underresponsive children have difficulty recognizing these states at all and may not be able to tell when they feel hungry, thirsty, hot, or cold, are excited, or need to use the restroom.

Many of these children, on both sides of the coin, benefit from a firm daily schedule, which may be thought of as an exposure. A reliable routine can be set for daily events such as meals, snacks, bathroom use, and bedtime. Parents are able to set the portion size for snacks and meals, particularly when the children are young. In this way, parents are helping their child to make appropriate decisions regarding when and how much to eat and drink. The same is true for elimination: a daily schedule should be set for using the restroom. Every morning the child should sit on the toilet for at least 20 minutes to try to void his bowels. Children who are dysregulated in this area either do not recognize the need to void or do not like the process and avoid it altogether. Setting a regular schedule helps them to feel that voiding is predictable (avoiding accidents later in the day) and that it is "just a part of the day." Sensory interventions, such as playing with interesting toys, using a head massager, and listening to music, as well as coping skill such as relaxation, cognitive correction, and deep breathing can make the process less uncomfortable for the child. Having a schedule such as this helps to organize the environment and expectations, and helps to train the nervous system to expect to eliminate waste at certain times. Schedules for urination can help avoid accidents as well. Set a schedule for school that requires a trip to the restroom at 2-hour increments and right after school to ensure frequent opportunities to urinate. Coping skills can help children learn to manage and tolerate the internal senses and also be able to exert some control over these uncomfortable feelings. For example, relaxation training after doing jumping jacks can help a child who does not like having a fast heartbeat. Rewards for following the schedule both at home and at school can encourage motivation and commitment to therapy.

Vestibular

Children who are overresponsive to the vestibular sense may find movement unpleasant and therefore avoid places like playgrounds and amusement parks. These children often dislike climbing, swinging, sliding, riding in a car, and even swimming. By contrast, vestibular-underresponsive children crave movement and may spin, rock, run, and bounce from one piece of equipment to the next with little regard for appropriateness or safety.

Exposure may be beneficial for vestibular-overresponsive children. These children can start to engage in movement by joining a gymnastics class that builds on basic skills, such as walking in a straight line on a mat, and then move to a low balance beam, and so on. Practicing swinging on a swing set with increasing intensity (exposure) while listening to a favorite song or counting the number of pushes (counterconditioning) can help alleviate some of the discomfort. Sensory-seeking children also benefit from class activities such as gymnastics or swimming because they are structured and organized, allowing them to develop skills and learn safety rules, as well as lessons about sportsmanship and sharing.

Proprioceptive

Children who have challenges with the proprioceptive sense have difficulty knowing where their body is in relation to other objects. They can appear rigid, tense, inflexible, and awkward. They bump into objects, have poor coordination, and are challenged playing sports such as football, basketball, volleyball, and tennis.

Exposure in the form of a yoga class can be ideal for children with proprioceptive sensory dysregulation. These classes help the child learn how it feels to stretch their bodies, loosen rigid postures, and increase flexibility. In addition, a class atmosphere encourages fun, socialization, and camaraderie while challenging the proprioceptive sense. Once proprioceptive difficulties have been identified, parents should be cautioned about pushing their child into a sport that will be difficult for him, such as football, baseball, or soccer, at a young age. More appropriate sports such as karate, gymnastics, track, ballet, or yoga should be explored first to increase body awareness and provide exercise. Other, more challenging sports can be introduced later, once skills have been built.

CONCLUSION

This chapter has presented suggestions for successfully using exposure when treating children who have anxiety coupled with sensory dysregulation, with the assistance of sensory interventions, coping skills, counterconditioning, and the use of rewards. This is by no means an exhaustive list of the techniques that can be used to treat sensory dysregulation—rather, it is a starting point. Ideas deemed appropriate by the therapist should be utilized on a case-by-case basis when developing a comprehensive treatment plan. In some cases, referral to an occupational therapist is a good first step, as these professionals are trained in helping children address sensory-based issues.

The next chapter discusses the critical role that parents play in the treatment of children with anxiety coupled with sensory dys-regulation.

CHAPTER 7

The Challenging Child
in Context
Involving Parents in Treatment

Treating children with mental health issues almost always includes working with their parents in some capacity. Because children with sensory regulation issues can experience their biggest challenges in the context of their family, working with parents and siblings is an important part of treatment. Left untreated, these difficult behaviors cause a tremendous amount of tension for parents, and often for the entire family. This chapter provides an overview of the parent role in therapy and how best to utilize parents as a piece of the therapy puzzle.

ACCOMMODATING
INAPPROPRIATE BEHAVIORS

Accommodating behaviors include those that reinforce inappropriate behavior, often unintentionally. As part of the initial evaluation, it is important to gather information about how parents and other family members have responded to the child's behavior thus far. In other words, what reactions, punishments, consequences, and feedback have family members given the child as a result of her behavior? Typically, parents respond to anxiety with anxiety. Well-meaning parents often fall prey to their own anxieties and respond to their child's fearful behavior by accommodating (doing exactly what the child wants) to help relieve the anxiety. In a way, parents may feel like relieving anxiety is a part of their job as good parents. In an effort to feel effective parents will:

- Sleep with their child (or allow her to sleep in the parents' bed) to ensure a good night's sleep and soothe anxieties.
- Eliminate chores and responsibilities so as not to add too much stress for the child.
- Allow their anxious child to stay home from school for days or weeks to avoid the possibility of being upset at school.
- Be unwilling to set appropriate limits with a child due to a desire to keep the peace.
- Complete tasks for children (homework, projects, chores) to shield them from stress.
- Fail to impose consequences for inappropriate behavior for fear that symptoms may worsen.

Unfortunately, these parenting behaviors serve to accommodate, and thus reinforce, a child's anxiety. Allowing a child to benefit in some way from his anxious behavior actually reinforces the behavior. It is important to help parents recognize their own accommodating behaviors and address them directly. Often this requires that parents be willing to tolerate their own anxiety in the process, and separate sessions with parents may be needed in addition to the family or child sessions.

Start normalizing the behavior by explaining how common it is for parents to react in these ways because it is hard to watch your child suffer. Explain, however, that therapy will sometimes involve having the parents allow their child to endure difficult situations. Psychoeducation is as important for parents as it is for children. Help parents to understand that therapy is sometimes difficult and that the greater good is the health and flexibility of their child. Explain that their role is to be supporters and advocates, not rescuers and appeasers. During the course of therapy they may need to set limits, reduce or discontinue accommodating behaviors, or encourage their child to engage in challenging behaviors that were previously avoided. Often these parental actions do not feel good or soothing to a child, and the parents must be prepared for their child to react with anger, frustration, or increased anxiety.

> When Camille (the fifth grader from Chapter 1) began to develop a fear of thunderstorms, her mother would lie in bed and comfort her. This quickly progressed to Camille wanting to lie down and be cuddled during cloudy days. Eventually, Camille would only sleep in her parents' bed, refused to sleep over at a friend's house, and threw tantrums when her parents discussed taking a trip without her. Despite all of this extra love, attention, and soothing, Camille's anxiety grew, and her ability to control and manipulate the family was causing problems in her parents' marriage.

Therapy for Camille and her family would involve Camille moving toward sleeping in her own bed, alone. This might be done with a behavior chart that allotted rewards for solo sleeping or it might be done in a graduated manner, where her parents spend less and less time with her before bedtime until she is able to face sleeping alone. It would be normal and expected for Camille to dislike either of these approaches and to argue that she could not sleep by herself. Starting exposure on a weekend or over the summer vacation might help reduce parental fears about Camille not sleeping and being tired at school. If that is not possible, the parents would have to accept the fact that Camille might have a few restless nights and tired days. Preparing parents for difficult times and discussing how to handle specific situations—for example, "Camille tried to sneak into our bed during the night" or "Camille screamed for 2 hours before falling asleep"—might be helpful to prevent her parents from getting surprised and anxiously falling back into old habits.

> THERAPIST: You are going to try some new things this weekend, Camille. We talked about how it is scary for you to sleep in your own bed, especially when you are alone and even more so if it is stormy outside.
>
> CAMILLE: Yes, I cannot sleep alone, especially if there is a storm. I will not sleep at all if they don't let me sleep with them. I do not think that it is a good idea at all.

THERAPIST: Well, I know that it feels like it would be very hard or even impossible, but I also think that you will be much happier when you are able to sleep in your own bed and you can spend the night with your friends. Your parents and I talked about how you could earn rewards for staying the whole night in your own bed. Mom, what do you think?

MOM: Dad and I thought that you could earn points for each night that you sleep in your own bed. When you earn enough points, maybe you could earn that phone you have been hoping to get before middle school.

CAMILLE: I could get a cell phone? Now, what would I have to do? Sleep in my own bed? I might be willing to do that, but only if I can get a phone.

THERAPIST: You would have to work out with your parents how many points it would take to earn the phone, but I usually recommend that you have at least 30 successes to earn the reward. You could earn the reward in 1 month or in 1 year, it would be up to you.

CAMILLE: I think that I would try to do it in 1 month!

THERAPIST: In the beginning, in addition to earning points toward the phone, you may also earn a pancake breakfast when you sleep in your room by yourself.

CAMILLE: You mean I could start out by earning a point toward my phone *and* get pancakes for breakfast?

THERAPIST: Yes, for the first week, breakfast would be part of the reward. After that, you will still earn points toward getting your cell phone.

CAMILLE: Well, that sounds great!

THERAPIST: Sounds like you are excited about this plan, Camille. Now let's talk about some things that could happen in the beginning while you are working on this plan. In the beginning, it will be hard to spend the whole night by yourself because you are not used to it. You might ask your parents to change their mind and let you get into their bed, especially if it is raining. How will all of you handle this?

MOM: Well, what if she is really scared? What should we do?

THERAPIST: Great question, that will probably happen at some point. Camille, do you remember some of the things that you are supposed to do, your coping skills, when you are uncomfortable?

CAMILLE: Yes, I am supposed to do my deep breathing, listen to soft music, and remind myself that I am safe.

THERAPIST: Yes, that is perfect. Do you think that you can do this, instead of going into your parents' room?

CAMILLE: Yes, I think so.

THERAPIST: Mom, what will you do if Camille is upset and wants to come sleep with you and her father?

MOM: I suppose I will remind her to use her coping skills. But what if she is really upset and afraid?

THERAPIST: You may have to be strong and set limits with her. It is OK to comfort her briefly after you return her to her own bed or talk to her in her bed. This should be a very short conversation, though. Camille, remember when we talked about how things seem scarier at night, and then are OK in the morning?

CAMILLE: Yes.

THERAPIST: What if you write that down and you can read it to yourself when you are afraid?

CAMILLE: Yes, I will try that. I will also write a note about how much I want that cell phone!

INFLICTING HARSH PUNISHMENTS

Sometimes parents may take a less sympathetic approach and attempt to impose excessive discipline on a child who is truly suffering and struggling with sensory regulation. In an attempt to be good parents, they will:

- Scream, yell, and shame a child who is avoiding something (food, places, activities).
- Eliminate all sources of entertainment, including television,

phone, computer, or outings with friends, in order to "motivate" the child to be able to function better.

- Force their child to do things that he is avoiding, causing
  oppositional behavior or even depression.

Eight-year-old Brad, from Chapter 1, would not eat food that
was touching other food on his plate. His parents enforced the
family rule: you eat what is served or you don't eat at all. As a
result, Brad did not eat. After he had missed dinner for nearly 2
weeks in a row, his parents started taking away other privileges
due to concern about possible weight loss or malnutrition. They
began to restrict his screen time (no TV or computer) unless
Brad ate his dinner from one plate. Brad remained steadfast in
his refusal to eat at dinnertime unless his food was presented
on separate plates. Unfortunately, with his pleasurable activities being eliminated, he had no source of relaxation or pleasure
and became more frustrated, resentful, and withdrawn.

Many times parents are behaving the way their parents did with
them, or they are trying to help their children by providing a strict
family structure and consequences for what they deem to be bad
behavior. Unfortunately, both the use of harsh punishments and
accommodating unwanted behaviors (as described earlier) are
equally ineffective parenting styles. Children often end up feeling
more anxious, depressed, and misunderstood as a result of these
parenting styles.

Setting up a therapeutic program for a child, with the help
of her parents, can solve many of these problems. The family as
a whole should be made aware of the goals of therapy, the behavior plan for each week, and appropriate reactions to behaviors that
will likely occur. It is the job of the therapist to expressly outline
how the therapy program will work so that inappropriate reactions
(such as harsh punishments) will not take place. Most important
is to teach parents how to positively reinforce appropriate behaviors, both verbally and with concrete rewards. As discussed in
Chapter 5, setting up a reinforcement/reward schedule is imperative when working with children who have sensory sensitivities.
Parents have the role of encouraging appropriate behaviors and
not accommodating inappropriate ones. Furthermore, the role of

parents changes dramatically from one developmental stage to the next. The following section describes typical functioning for each stage of childhood development and how sensory dysregulation can impact the family system, as well as how to manage these issues at each developmental stage.

SENSORY DYSFUNCTION ACROSS DEVELOPMENTAL STAGES

0–2 Years

It is helpful to understand the tasks children face at each developmental stage before beginning to treat a child with sensory regulation issues. The developmental experience for babies (ages 0–2) includes inability to communicate needs, limited environment (stays in crib), unable to identify or independently meet needs for food, rest, stimulation, or mobility, and limited means of coping. Sensory dysregulation at this early developmental stage can undermine the confidence of parents because they feel as if they cannot effectively meet the most basic needs of their child. Specifically, these babies are not able to be soothed, seem inconsolable, are in constant discomfort, cry incessantly, and appear to be unhappy most of the time, despite great efforts from parents to soothe and comfort their young child. In addition, parents may get subtle or overt messages from grandparents and friends that they are doing something wrong to cause the distress.

Sensory dysregulation in the very young child can greatly impact his parents; it can interrupt the establishment of a daily routine, disrupt family life, and sometimes cause marital discord. This can be an extremely difficult and stressful time for parents and families. Intervention at this early stage provides an excellent opportunity to assist a family in crisis. Parent coping can be improved if instead of blaming themselves, parents gain a better understanding of the source of their child's distress. They can also learn to soothe their child in unconventional ways so that the baby is relieved of his discomfort and learns to soothe himself. Some unconventional ways to soothe an inconsolable child with sensory dysregulation include:

- Tight swaddling and less human touch, which can provide a nice break from stimulation.
- Placing the child in a car seat on top of a running clothes dryer, which provides sensory vibrations that some children find comforting.
- Leaving the vacuum cleaner turned on near the child. The constant humming sound can be soothing to some children.
- Having the parent strap the child into a wearable carrier—a snuggle sack, for example—while the parent walks around the house completing tasks. The warmth and movement of the parent can be soothing to the child.

2–5 Years

Toddlers gain certain skills as part of their developmental stage: verbal skills, some coping skills, the ability to expand their environment (i.e., moving out of a crib and into a bed, becoming more mobile), and an emerging ability to identify their need for food, rest, and stimulation. Babies who have sensory dysregulation may, without assistance, grow into toddlers with the same problem who continue to greatly disrupt family life. Toddlers who are overreactive will exhibit meltdowns, temper tantrums, hitting, and biting and be unwilling to participate in age-appropriate activities. Grandparents, friends, and even strangers can be eager to offer parenting advice, often implying that the child is misbehaving due to poor parenting. These well-meaning suggestions undermine an already fragile confidence, leading parents to feel ineffective at managing their own children.

Underreactive 2- to 5-year-old children who seek stimulation may often engage in bizarre behaviors such as licking, smelling, and touching inappropriately, causing embarrassment and shame for many parents. Whereas parents may feel completely helpless and confused about why their baby is inconsolable, during the toddler years children are more able to verbalize their discomfort. In a way, it is easier because parents are somewhat aware of what is bothering their child, but they are often mistaken about why it is bothering him. In other words, a child might be able to verbalize "I hate hairbrushes!" but is not able to explain, "It feels like you are stabbing my scalp with toothpicks when you brush my hair and I cannot stand the pain!" For this reason, avoidant or resistant behavior at this age gets classified as "terrible twos" or oppositional when, in fact, it may have a sensory genesis.

The therapist can be very helpful in restoring a sense of confidence and competence in parents of young children. It is important to provide information about the sensory nervous system, telling parents how sensitivities or differences in the nervous system can impact behavior and what they can do to help their child function, given her sensory differences. Simply thinking "It is not my fault" and "My child has some differences that are causing these disturbances in behavior" can help parents to develop empathy for their child and move toward responding differently.

Very young children are highly reliant on their parents to get their most basic needs met. Parents determine when and what to eat, what to wear, when to sleep, and in what type of activities to participate. The world of the young child largely revolves around the parent. Therefore, when working with very young children who have sensory regulation issues, parents are extremely involved in treatment. As with potty training, the parent is the important factor in facilitating behavior change in the home. Parents are asked to monitor their child's behavior as well as their own reactions to the behavior. The therapist will help identify the relevant antecedents to the behavior, the behavior itself, and the consequences, as well as behavioral accommodations (as noted above) and any secondary reinforcing behaviors that are occurring. Parents are given ample information to help them understand the child's behavior within the context of his nervous system and how the behavior is maintained by the family interactions. Finally, parents and the therapist will explore interventions to help improve coping, enhance the child's sensory comfort, discourage the child's avoidant behavior, and create a reward system in order to facilitate tolerating sensory input.

5–11 Years

Typical development for this age includes increasing contact with the outside world beyond the family. Children begin to forge their own relationships with peers and with nonfamily adults. This stage is also referred to as the age of industry because children are acquiring academic, athletic, musical, and social skills. They begin to compare themselves to others scholastically, socially, and economically. This developmental stage is also the age of onset for troubles with learning differences, ADHD, Tourette syndrome, anxiety disorders, and increased stress due to expectations at school.

When children in this stage of development present for treatment of anxiety but have comorbid sensory regulation issues, their behavior is often marked by noncompliance, frequent tantrums, or abrupt meltdowns. These and other avoidant behaviors (avoidance of loud parties, or going to the beach or an amusement park) can impact peer relationships, academics, and/or relationships with important adults such as teachers. Teachers may also contact the family with concerns regarding the child's behavior, such as being unwilling to go outside for recess, difficulty completing basic work assignments for fear of making a mistake, or oppositional, rigid behavior.

Treatment for the elementary-school-age child requires parent and child to become a team. As always, begin by providing valuable information about sensory dysregulation, but this time the information will be directed at team members. This allows the child and parent to develop a better understanding of the challenging behaviors being experienced and discussed in treatment. Learning about the nervous system and how this sensitive system interacts with the child's behavior can help facilitate empathy toward the child and encourage an alliance between the child and her parents. The therapist can then encourage and assist in the development of a well-designed incentive system to encourage maximum participation in treatment.

> THERAPIST: Can you tell me the difficulties that Courtney is having in her second-grade class at school?
>
> PARENT: Yes. Courtney gets easily upset at school. She is a bright girl, but when the teacher asks the class to write anything down, Courtney starts to cry and get angry. She says that she can't write as fast as the other children and when she tries, she makes mistakes. Courtney's explosions at school are really annoying the teacher and the other children. Even

kids who used to be her friends are not playing with her any longer because they don't like her crying and throwing things all the time. Courtney has always been a sensitive child. As a toddler she was pretty controlling and needed to have things in her room exactly right. She told others where to sit and would even rearrange the placemats on the table so that she could have the same one at each meal. We always thought it was a phase and that she would grow out of it. But she seems to have taken this need for perfection to school, and it is really affecting her relationships with her peers and her teacher.

THERAPIST: That sounds really hard. So Courtney is having trouble tolerating imperfection, is having frequent crying episodes, and is losing her friends. That must be terrible for you too.

PARENT: Oh, it is! My husband and I are constantly talking about what to do about Courtney. My husband thinks she needs to pull herself up by her bootstraps and stop being so dramatic. I think she is suffering and needs more attention. I am exhausted trying to find fun things for Courtney to do with me, since she doesn't have any friends right now. My husband is really mad at me because he thinks I am making the situation worse.

THERAPIST: Tension at home is very common when these situations come up. Let's talk about what is likely driving this behavior and how to find some common ground.

PARENT: That is exactly what we are looking for.

THERAPIST: It sounds as if Courtney has anxiety about perfection. She seems to be unable to tolerate imperfection in many forms. Sometimes this behavior is driven by having a sensitive nervous system. We receive many forms of sensory input throughout the day. Our nervous system collects that information, interprets it, and then determines how best to respond. When there is an emergency, our nervous system informs us by producing a fight, flight, or freeze response. When a person has a sensitive nervous system, some of that sensory information is interpreted inaccurately, and the

response is fight, flight, or freeze even when there is no crisis. This feeling is pretty awful, so these children quickly
develop irritable reactions or controlling behaviors in order
to try to avoid that awful feeling. Children may be anxious
about seeing something that will upset them, such as not
having the right placemat, or producing something that is
not up the their standards, such as a writing assignment at
school.

PARENT: Yes, that's it. She would have huge meltdowns if someone was sitting at "her" seat at the kitchen table. This was
particularly embarrassing when my friends would come
over for a cup of coffee and Courtney would see that "her"
seat was taken, even if she was playing in another room. She
would scream, cry, and throw things.

THERAPIST: This is a good example of a sensitive nervous system and overresponse to seeing something that, in her mind,
is out of place. Unfortunately, this overreactive response
results in negative reactions from those around her, so not
only is she internally irritable and upset, the people in her
environment are also pretty unhappy and frustrated.

PARENT: That sounds like exactly what is happening.

THERAPIST: The good news is that we can develop a treatment
plan to help Courtney and you cope with her sensitivities.
The first step is to help Courtney understand more about
anxiety and how her unique nervous system works. This
will allow her to understand why she sometimes feels so
upset. Then we will discuss a variety of skills to help Courtney learn to tolerate her anxious feelings and at the same
time soothe her nervous system. We can even build in some
rewards for practicing her new skills. Let's have Courtney
come with you for the next session.

12–17 Years

Adolescence is typically a tumultuous stage for any child and her
family. Normal development includes academic tasks such as

abstract thinking, increasing scholastic demands, and beginning to plan for the future. Social features entail the beginning of separating from the family, increased autonomy, and identity formation. Adolescents start to value their peers' opinions above those of the family. Teenagers emerge as sexual beings, beginning to identify sexual orientation and making decisions about becoming sexually active. Adolescence is also the time for the onset of depression, bipolar disorder, OCD, panic disorder, generalized anxiety disorder, social phobia, specific phobia, eating disorders, substance abuse issues, and some psychotic disorders. More than anything, adolescence is a time for rebellion and conflict with parents, ranging from mild belligerence to severe acting out.

Adolescents who are functioning normally still exhibit characteristics of separation and individuation (defiance, being obstinate, talking back). When sensory dysregulation is also present, it can significantly impair academic, social, and family functioning. In addition, these adolescents have typically suffered for years without understanding why they feel the way they do. Years of stubborn, well-practiced habits make behavior change more difficult to achieve. Parents, too, have engaged in years of reacting with frustration or accommodation, or have simply given up on the belief that their child's behavior can change. Sometimes just understanding their adolescent's nervous system and realizing why he has been avoiding and resisting for so many years can be an "Aha" experience that opens to door to healing. Psychoeducation is perhaps the most powerful intervention at this stage because it answers so many previously unanswered questions. Parents' reactions to this information can be relief (that someone finally understands their child), disbelief (that something so physiological can explain what they always assumed to be willful and the result of bad behavior), or guilt (that they have so profoundly misunderstood and blamed their child for all of these years). Adolescents tend to react with relief (that they are finally understood), anger, or "I told you so" reactions toward their parents.

The therapist should forge an independent relationship with the adolescent during treatment. Parents should be minimally involved, which, for some, can be challenging. It may be helpful for parents to participate in their own treatment to help confront their own anxieties and develop healthy ways to disengage from being enmeshed with or overly reactive to their teenage child. The teen and therapist may determine that periodic updates with the parents might be helpful. Parents may benefit from becoming more attuned to looking for new, healthy, and sometimes subtle behaviors that are being displayed at home by the adolescent. In this way parents can reinforce the exposure behaviors and use of sensory interventions and notice when sensory stimuli are being well tolerated.

PARENTING AT EVERY STAGE

At each stage of development, parents should be informed about normal development and about how anxiety and sensory dysregulation can impact functioning. Parent involvement varies depending on the child's age and developmental stage.

Parents of children at any stage benefit from being reminded of certain basic cognitive- behavioral principles (e.g., any attention can be reinforcing). When a child is engaging in a dysfunctional behavior, and her parent yells, gets upset, or comforts her, the dysfunctional behavior may be reinforced. This is a difficult concept for many parents and important for them to understand.

Most parents pay more attention to children's unwanted behaviors and ignore desirable behaviors. This is exactly the opposite of what therapy hopes to accomplish. Parents end up reinforcing those maladaptive behaviors, and the adaptive behaviors go unrewarded. Introducing the concept of differential reinforcement can be extremely useful. Help parents to understand that they can reinforce, or pay more attention to, the desired behaviors and less attention to the other behaviors. This will help reduce maladaptive behaviors and reinforce those that are more functional.

Another important principle to remind parents about is the extinction burst. Parents believe that if they ignore a behavior, it will immediately go away. That is not true. There can be an increase (burst) of the behavior first before it becomes extinct. Therefore, parents must be prepared for and anticipate this phenomenon if they are to be successful using ignoring as a technique.

HELPING PARENTS DEVELOP EMPATHY

Unless a child is adopted, and therefore not the biological child of the parents, almost always one of the parents also experienced some sensory dysregulation while growing up. It is helpful early in treatment to explore parents' understanding of their own nervous systems to help them to get a clearer picture of what their child is dealing with. Asking questions about their own history or having a parent ask his parents about his own history as a child is a great way to start. Normalizing sensory experiences by providing common examples can also help a parent understand these concepts.

> THERAPIST: Mr. Johnson, tell me what you were like as a child—did you have any special likes or dislikes, such as loud noises, smells, tastes, or textures?

> MR. JOHNSON: Well, nothing like Sally, but I did hate it when my mother would brush my hair, and I could not stand it when I flushed the toilet, it scared the heck out of me. But that is different from Sally, she flat-out refuses to wear socks and only eats five types of food.

> THERAPIST: Actually, it really is very much the same thing. What did you do when you had to flush the toilet? I am curious.

> MR. JOHNSON: I would flush it and run! It scared me so bad that at night I would just leave it and wait to flush it in the morning. And my mom just let me wear my hair like a mop. I looked like a ragamuffin half the time, but I didn't care.

> THERAPIST: So you see, you and Sally are a lot alike. Those dislikes and fears may be different from hers, but they are all sensory based. As a kid, what would it have felt like to you if you were forced to have your hair brushed every morning, or if you were made to flush the toilet and stand there while it flushed? That is pretty much what you are doing to her when you make her wear socks every day or force her to eat foods that she can't tolerate. Now, there are other ways to help Sally be able to tolerate these sensory experiences, but we have to go about it a little differently.

MR. JOHNSON: Wow, I feel like I owe her an apology. I did not understand what she has been feeling. Tell me what I need to do.

AVOIDING SHAME

There is a huge difference between guilt and shame when parenting a child. Guilt might result from a statement such as "You are a great kid, but what you just did was not a great decision" versus a shame-inducing statement such as "I am so disappointed in you." One statement avoids the internalization of the bad choice, and the other promotes the internalization of badness. When working with parents, it is very important to make sure that they are not using shame-inducing statements, especially when they have a child with sensory-based issues. Many times these children are particularly sensitive to criticism and even more vulnerable to internalization of the negative. Role-play with parents how to respond to their child's behaviors and model appropriate responses in session. It is helpful to keep the focus on choices and consequences, rather than worthiness. Here is an example of a conversation among parent, child, and therapist:

PEARSON: I had a really hard time yesterday, I was disgusted by the sticky feeling on my fingers and I lost it. I yelled at the party, and my mom had to take me out screaming. I felt really sad afterward and like I was a really bad person.

PARENT: Yes, it was awful. Pearson just started freaking out. I tried to get him to wash his hands, but he flat-out refused. I was so upset and embarrassed. I was mortified and we just left. I am sure we will never get invited back there again, right, Pearson?

THERAPIST: Hang on a minute. So Pearson felt bad that he had a sticky feeling on his fingers and started to react to it. Is that right?

PEARSON: Yes.

THERAPIST: So you made a choice to not wash your hands, is that what you did?

PEARSON: Yes, I guess so.

THERAPIST: OK, looking back on it, can you think of another thing that you could have done instead?

PEARSON: Well, I could have washed my hands, but I really do not like the bathroom at that kid's house, it has a really funky smell in it and I don't like going in there.

THERAPIST: OK, so are there other options for washing your hands there?

PEARSON: I guess I could have done it in the kitchen, or used a wet wipe. They had wet wipes at the party. I was just mad at my mom for the way she was talking to me, it made me even more mad.

THERAPIST: So, you made a choice that did not work for you, but you know that next time you have the ability to make a different choice. Pearson, you responded when your nervous system was telling you that you were in danger, but you were really just uncomfortable. Mom, it sounds like you could have made a different choice as well. How could you have reacted differently to Pearson's predicament?

PARENT: Well, I could have helped him problem-solve how to get the stickiness off of his hands instead of yelling at him. I just get so frustrated when he loses it.

THERAPIST: If you think about it, you and Pearson are a lot alike. You both react quickly when you are uncomfortable with the situation. Maybe you can both work on recognizing when this is happening and help each other out, more like a team.

It is always important to stress to parents the importance of not reacting with shame statements, sticking to problem solving, and avoiding reacting with negative emotion.

SUCCESS IN TREATMENT

Parents will always be involved to a certain degree in the treatment of children, particularly those with sensory regulation issues.

Expectations should be set early, stating that therapy involves work for all parties involved. In fact, most of the work occurs outside of the therapy office. Metaphors such as learning to play the piano can be helpful. The instructor can give the lesson, but if the student does not practice between lessons, the student's piano skills will not improve. Like piano, practice between sessions is imperative for success in treatment.

CONCLUSION

This chapter has outlined parents' role in treatment, from being highly involved with very young children to less involved, if at all, with the older adolescent. Parents of school-age children participate a great deal in treatment alongside their child, forming a team. Therapy should focus on increasing empathy, avoiding shame, and improving the parent–child connection. When parents are appropriately and actively involved in treatment for children of any age with sensory dysregulation, the result is improved family functioning and lifelong positive change.

CHAPTER 8

Integrating Treatment for Sensory Dysregulation into Therapy for Specific Disorders

While the previous seven chapters have reviewed how sensory dysregulation impacts childhood behavior and psychological functioning, this chapter details case presentations of children who present with common disorders but have underlying sensory dysregulation as a driving force. As stated previously, the treatment formula is somewhat different for children who have sensory-based issues because, in these types of cases, traditional exposure therapy is not sufficient. Treatment for cases of OCD, generalized anxiety disorder, specific phobia, social phobia, oppositional defiant disorder, and compulsive skin picking will be outlined in detail utilizing the treatment formula specific to sensory dysregulation: Exposure + Sensory Intervention + Coping Skills + Counterconditioning = Tolerance for the sensory stimulus.

OBSESSIVE–COMPULSIVE DISORDER

Chad is a 14-year-old freshman in high school. He has always had a need to have his room orderly, but this year his need for neatness has affected his ability to function at school. In middle school Chad could not settle down to complete his homework unless his work space was completely clear and his pencils and pens were all lined up neatly. He would empty his backpack, spend 15–20 minutes setting up his work area, and then get started on his homework. When he had a question, one of his parents would sit with him, answer his question, and discuss the homework. Although Chad found the discussion helpful, he always felt the need to straighten up and reorder his surroundings after his parent left. This often took another 20 to 30 minutes before he could resume his work. Chad's need for a neat work space seemed limited to home and did not affect his functioning at school.

When Chad entered high school, his need for a neat desk at school began to interfere with his ability to complete his schoolwork. Chad became very anxious until his desk in each class was cleared off, his pens and pencils lined up, and his papers neatly displayed. This often took Chad 15 minutes or so, just as it did when he was home working on his homework. Due to the time it took to settle in, Chad often missed the first part of each lesson in all of his classes. He fell behind quickly. Chad would also get upset and combative when a teacher urged him to hurry and catch up to the rest of the class.

Chad's parents saw their bright, previously excellent student begin to fail the majority of his ninth-grade classes. In addition, Chad became argumentative and angry with teachers and other students, further isolating himself from others. This is when Chad's parents brought him in to therapy for help.

Step 1: Make the Diagnosis and Provide Education

At the onset of treatment it was important for Chad's therapist to determine if he was treating OCD or sensory dysregulation that looked a lot like OCD. A key question for a case of OCD in particular is "What would happen if you did not clear off your work space?" Chad and his therapist discussed what it was like for Chad when he saw his environment looking, in his view, cluttered or in disarray. Chad described feeling uncomfortable when he saw messes around his work area, stating that they looked wrong and made his heart race and his stomach tighten. His discomfort was so significant that he had to clean up his work space in order to feel comfortable and concentrate on his work. Eventually, he became focused on creating the perfect, clean work space to avoid these uncomfortable physical feelings. Never once did Chad report that something bad would happen or a negative outcome would result (other than not being able to gain comfort) if he did not participate in this ritual. Instead, he described uncomfortable physical experiences that were bothersome to him, and wanting to avoid them. This is key questioning for a case such as this, as it helps to highlight what factors are driving the behavior. As is the case with OCD, he started to avoid or alter situations that led to anxiety or discomfort, but the source of the discomfort was different. In this case, the source of the discomfort was "the way it looks," not "If I don't do this, something bad will happen to me or someone else." Asking the questions provided in Chapter 3 about sensory dysregulation and childhood history of sensory processing issues can also illuminate these issues. That said, Chad's treatment still involved exposure and response prevention (ERP), with the addition of the other important interventions that target dysregulation, because the source of his discomfort was sensory and lacked an obsessional theme.

Psychoeducation was provided to both Chad and his parents regarding his nervous system and, more specifically, his particular sensitivities. Mom and Dad reported that Chad had been a difficult baby, hard to console and easily agitated. They also described a host of other sensory sensitivities he has faced during his development, further confirming the hypothesis that he has a dysregulated nervous system.

Step 2: Create an Exposure Hierarchy

Chad's need for neatness was discussed, and a hierarchy was created identifying 10 steps, from least troublesome to most anxiety provoking, to slowly and systematically expose him to increasingly messy environments, thus increasing his tolerance for them:

1. Do homework with a few pencils out of place.
2. Do homework with pencils and pens out of place.
3. Do homework with pencils, pens, and a paper in disarray.
4. Do homework with pencils, pens, and papers in disarray, and with his backpack on the table.
5. Do work in school with pencils out of place.
6. Do work in school with pencils and pens out of place.

7. Do work in school with pencils, pens, and paper in disarray.

8. Do work in school with pencils, pens, papers, and text-
   books in disarray.

9. Do work in school with no extra supplies out and work with
   disheveled papers, a textbook, and a single pen or pencil.

10. Work at home in a room that is in disarray, on a table with
    few supplies, which are disorganized and out of place.

Chad felt this hierarchy captured the circumstances that would increase his discomfort. He understood that he would work his way up the hierarchy, challenging himself with progressively more uncomfortable tasks while managing his anxiety along the way.

Step 3: Teach Sensory Interventions

Sensory interventions were added to help Chad soothe his nervous system while he simultaneously worked on exposures. His therapist explained that he would be better able to tolerate those challenging situations by tending to his internal system. After trying many different sensory strategies across the five senses during a therapy session, Chad and his therapist selected several interventions and made a plan. In order to soothe his nervous system, Chad decided to try some sensory distractions that also provided soothing sensory input to distract him from the visual chaos of his environment. At school he decided to try:

- Carrying smooth stones in his pockets and rubbing his fin-
  gers on them.
- Squeezing a stress ball.
- Chewing cinnamon gum.

At home he made a plan to get some exercise right after school to release some of his stress from the day. He reported that exercise had a calming effect on him. In addition to some of the tactile interventions he selected for school, he would add some other interventions that would not be possible at school, such as playing with Silly

Putty, rubbing pipe cleaners between his fingers, lighting a eucalyptus candle in his homework area, as this is his favorite scent, playing classical music softly while he did homework, and wrapping himself in a soft blanket that he uses when he sleeps. He stated that he associates the blanket with relaxation and feeling calm.

Step 4: Teach Coping Skills

Chad's therapist introduced relaxation training. Chad learned how deep breathing can relax his body in a variety of situations and also help him fall asleep. He also learned how to do progressive muscle relaxation while sitting at a desk. His homework was to practice using the relaxation strategies before going to bed, before school, and before starting his homework. Chad also created a list of coping statements that helped him remember he was developing new skills to help him with anxiety. These coping statements reminded Chad that each time he felt anxious was an opportunity to practice using his coping skills. The coping statements that Chad developed were:

> "I have a sensitive nervous system, so I may feel upset when I see things out of place."
> "I can manage my nervous system."
> "I can practice deep breathing."
> "Everybody feels anxious sometimes."
> "Anxiety gives me a chance to practice my skills."
> "I will get better at using my skills the more I practice them."

Chad began to read these statements and added to the list as time went along. Another coping skill was to use a mindfulness technique. Chad was asked to sit with the messy desk and simply describe how it looked. He would take 5–10 minutes and describe in detail (either out loud or by writing on paper) what the mess looked like, without judging it as wrong or bad. In addition, he was asked to describe how he was feeling internally while observing the mess—for example, "My stomach is tight," "My breathing is fast," or "My heart is beating rapidly." This intervention helped him to see the mess as something to observe and describe, rather than something to fix. After he was done describing the mess, he could then start his homework.

Step 5: Incorporate Counterconditioning

After much discussion, a counter conditioning idea was developed. Chad's mom would cover his desk with brightly wrapped candies. He was to complete his homework in the "mess" and then clean up by eating the candy. Chad liked this idea, and it was added to the treatment plan.

Step 6: Institute a Reward System

A reward system was added to the treatment plan. Chad would earn a reward for practicing his new skills and using them during exposures. Each time Chad practiced using his skills while doing exposures, he could earn money so that he could buy a new camera. He and his parents agreed that $2 a day could be earned for practice. Chad's parents were reminded to always accompany the tangible reward with a positive verbal comment such as "You did a great job using your deep breathing while completing your homework" or "Nice work using coping statements before starting your homework."

Instituting a reward system can be tricky. Chad felt the best reward for him would be money, and his parents agreed to the use of money and the amount. Each family and child is different in terms of the amount of money and the items they find reinforcing. The reward must be reinforcing to the child and not punishing to the parents (e.g., $100 a day for practice or a new car at the end of the month). Rewards that are unrealistic or too difficult to earn do not encourage enduring behavior change. It's very important to work with the child and the parents to find a suitable reward that is both appropriate and manageable over time.

Step 7: Implement a Comprehensive Treatment Plan

Chad's treatment plan began with reading coping statements each evening before bed and each morning while eating breakfast. In addition, Chad practiced his deep breathing skills and progressive muscle relaxation before bed. Chad practiced these skills each day for 1 week. Every morning Chad would fill out a chart indicating whether or not he had read the coping statements, practiced deep breathing, and practiced progressive muscle relaxation skills the night before. In addition, Chad would mark the chart for the morning, showing if had reviewed the coping statements. At the end of the day, Chad's mother would present him with his reward. A fully completed chart would earn $2, while a chart that was more than half complete would earn $1.

After 1 week, Chad added the use of sensory interventions to his plan and his chart. He was to use Silly Putty and pipe cleaners and listen to classical music while doing his homework. At school, Chad brought some smooth stones in his pockets and rubbed them while settling down to work. In addition, he began to practice observing his messy environment and his physical reaction to his messy environment while using deep breathing and sensory input. He practiced this for 5 minutes in places both at home and at school where there was no expectation that he would complete homework (a messy area in the family room, and while sitting in the cafeteria or in the classroom before the lesson began).

The chart grew with more interventions, and the family continued to use the same reward criteria, with a fully completed chart earning $2, and half or more complete earning $1. After 3 weeks, Chad noticed that not only was his anxiety more manageable, but he had also earned $35. He was eager to begin working his way up his exposure hierarchy.

Chad started his exposures at Step 3 because he felt that he could manage this and it would be a good, challenging place to start. Chad read his coping statements, practiced his deep breathing, and used his Silly Putty while doing his homework with pens or pencils and papers strewn around the work area. Chad's mother also threw some brightly wrapped candy around the table.

Chad discovered that he could complete his homework in a timely fashion, and as a result, his confidence grew and he was excited about working on more difficult exposures. Chad, his parents, and his therapist followed the treatment plan (Exposure + Sensory Intervention + Coping Skills + Counterconditioning =

Tolerance for the sensory stimulus), using the information developed during the early stages of therapy.

Chad felt confident completing his homework successfully and efficiently, and was able to manage his discomfort about having a messy work space. He decided that he wanted to jump ahead on the hierarchy and work on developing good skills at school as well as home. He started working on tolerating pens, pencils, and papers in disarray on his desk at school (level 7 on the hierarchy). Chad took deep breaths, reviewed his coping statements, chewed gum, and rubbed his fingers on smooth stones in his pockets while at school. He discovered that the practice at home made a significant difference in his ability to manage anxiety in the school setting as well.

As illustrated in this case example, utilizing the expanded treatment intervention for children with sensory dysregulation as the driving force behind their anxiety is the key to successful treatment. The formula can be used with a variety of different anxiety and psychological disorders, as will be demonstrated in the remainder of this chapter.

GENERALIZED ANXIETY DISORDER

Rachel is 10 years old and, according to her mother, is afraid of everything. She doesn't like trying new things, has difficulty with transitions, hates thunderstorms, doesn't want to attend sleepovers at friends' or relatives' homes, won't wear new clothes, won't go to places where she has not been before, is often irritable, and has difficulty sleeping. She seems upset much of the time, and her parents cannot seem to help settle her when she becomes agitated.

Rachel reports that she is upset by the thought of any new experiences because she does not know how they will feel. If there is any unknown experience presented to her, regardless of how exciting and fun it may be, she will refuse to participate. Her parents are frustrated and confused by her absolute refusal to shop for new clothes, visit new places, or participate in a variety of seemingly fun activities. In addition, due to Rachel's difficulty falling asleep, she does not want to sleep anywhere else but home, which makes family (and parent) travel virtually impossible.

Step 1: Make the Diagnosis and Provide Education

Rachel's therapist discovered that something other than anxiety was driving her avoidant behavior when she interviewed Rachel and her parents. Rachel's parents described her as being a very sensitive child, particularly to touch. She only wore certain clothes, hated to have her hair brushed, and clung to her soft blanket her entire childhood. After further questioning, it became apparent that Rachel has struggled with a variety of sensory sensitivities that have led her to avoid experiences where she must confront something that is new and unknown. This avoidance became a habit over the years and evolved into a generalized anxiety disorder where she worries about all new situations, fearing that she will have to confront some unpleasant sensory experience.

Step 2: Create an Exposure Hierarchy

An exposure hierarchy was created identifying 10 steps that involved facing progressively harder activities but incorporated activities that Rachel would enjoy as well.

1. Try eating a new type of candy.
2. Go to a new shopping center.
3. Try a new food at dinner.
4. Sleep in the guest room at home.
5. Go to the zoo.
6. Sleep in a sleeping bag in the family room.
7. Go on a day trip to a nearby theme park and eat food available at the park.
8. Sleep at her grandparents' house.
9. Go on a weekend trip to the beach with her family.
10. Sleep at a friend's house.

Step 3: Teach Sensory Interventions

Through discussion and trial and error, Rachel learned that certain sensory sensations helped her to feel calm. Interventions using these sensations included stroking satin material, hugging her soft blanket from childhood, doodling or drawing, and listening to her favorite country music. Rachel and her parents agreed to procure the items she did not already have and begin to use them around the house.

Step 4: Teach Coping Skills

Rachel was taught breathing retraining, and she practiced this for several weeks. She also developed a list of coping statements reminding her that she had a sensitive nervous system and that her upset feelings sometimes were simply error messages. Rachel also practiced using encouraging statements such as "I have always wanted to go to the zoo, this might really be fun" or "I will be so proud of myself when I am able to . . . [go to the zoo, sleep at a friend's house, try new food, etc.]." Furthermore, she practiced statements directed at anxiety about sleeping: "Even if I don't sleep, resting is also good for my body" and "I have been tired before and able to function the next day." These statements helped Rachel focus on developing good anxiety management skills rather than using avoidance to escape from the anxiety.

Step 5: Incorporate Counterconditioning

Rachel and her therapist created a "game" she could play while taking part in novel activities. While at the zoo, Rachel could keep track of all the different animals she might see, hoping to reach one hundred. While spending time with her grandparents at the mall, Rachel would count the number of times she heard the phrase "okie dokie artichokie," something they say frequently. Rachel would report the results of her observations to her therapist, and she would challenge herself to reach a higher number the next time she played the game.

Step 6: Institute a Reward System

To further assist with motivation and eliminate resistance, Rachel's parents agreed to establish a reward system. Rachel would earn points every day for using interventions and for working on her hierarchy. She decided to work for accessories for her American Girl dolls, and her parents agreed. She could earn small articles of clothing for her doll each day. When working with children, it is important that they earn small items early in the process. This helps them feel successful, builds confidence, and establishes commitment and motivation for the therapy process.

Step 7: Implement a Comprehensive Treatment Plan

Treatment for Rachel began with her actively practicing relaxation and deep breathing for several weeks while her family helped her gather the necessary sensory soothing items. She then started to practice engaging in exposure tasks while utilizing her coping statements, sensory interventions, and relaxation/deep breathing skills. Once she had conquered several low-level exposures, she gained confidence that she could do more difficult ones. She quickly worked up her hierarchy, feeling proud of herself for being able to do these tasks. Treatment gains were quite rapid, and Rachel was able to successfully sleep at a friend's house (a 10 on her hierarchy) within 6 weeks. She felt so confident with her new skills and abilities that she was excited to use her strategies and participate in many new situations.

SPECIFIC PHOBIA

Mary is a well-adjusted 10-year-old girl who recently started to avoid going to play at friends' houses. She stated that she doesn't like dogs and therefore won't go to anyone's house in case there is a dog there. Mary used to go to others' homes easily; however, a few months ago she went to a friend's house where there was a dog. The dog did not growl, bite, or jump on her, but it licked her, smelled her, and put its paws on her legs. She got extremely upset and had to leave. Since then, she has been unwilling to enter anyone else's home. After several months of coaxing, demanding, begging, and requiring her to visit relatives and friends, her parents brought her into treatment.

Step 1: Make the Diagnosis and Provide Education

Mary's parents were completely perplexed when they spoke with the therapist. As far as they knew, Mary had not been threatened in any way by that or any other dog. They guessed she was scared that the dog might try to hurt her, but she denied this. Mary's family had never owned a dog, and she had had limited interactions with this type of animal. Although she claims to love dogs, she has not really had much exposure to them.

During the first session, Mary's parents noted that she has always been a sensory-sensitive child. Mary could identify the type of soap her mom used to wash her hands and complained that certain foods smelled funny. She hated baths as a young child, not liking to be splashed or have her hair washed. She was one of the last children her age to learn how to swim because she did not like putting her face in the water. When Mary was younger she would only wear certain clothes that felt really soft and pleasing to her and avoided wearing clothes that were perceived to be rough, itchy, or too tight.

Mary told her therapist that she was not afraid of the dog, she just hated the way it smelled and couldn't stand the wet feeling on her arm or leg from the dog licking her or touching her with a wet nose. She always liked the idea of dogs, but when a dog got close to her and she could smell it, Mary immediately felt bad and wanted to leave. When the dog got even closer, she could feel its scratchy fur, which she said bothered her hands, and the slobber from the licking was more than she could take. She felt as if she had to get out of the house immediately.

Mary's early sensory sensitivities set the stage for her overreactivity to the dog's affectionate welcome. She was reacting with fear to her internal experience, not to the dog itself. The therapist explained how Mary's sensitive nervous system affected her current behavior.

Step 2: Create an Exposure Hierarchy

Mary really loved being with her friends and other family members. She missed being able to go to others' houses and play. Mary and her therapist started to create a hierarchy identifying 10 steps with progressively challenging behaviors based on Mary's discomfort with dogs:

1. Look at pictures of dogs or go to a dog park and view dogs at a distance from the car, while imagining being close to the dogs.
2. Same as 1, but get out of the car and walk close to dogs.
3. Same as 2, but pet a strange dog that is friendly (will have parents with her to evaluate for safety).
4. Sit in the therapist's office with a dog, but do not let it touch her in any way
5. Same as 4, but touch the dog in the office and pet the dog's body.
6. Same as 5, but also touch the dog's nose.
7. Same as 6, but allow the dog to put paws on her legs.
8. Same as 7, but also smell the dog and allow the dog to smell and lick her.
9. Go with her family to visit friends who do not own dogs.
10. Go to the house of a friend who has a dog for a play date.

Step 3: Teach Sensory Interventions

Once Mary understood the types of sensory input that upset her (unexpected touch that is scratchy, wet, or intense; strong dog smells), she was eager to explore different sensory experiences that would help soothe her. Mary discovered that she enjoyed quite a few different sensory items, such as smelling citrus-scented oils, sucking on hard candy with lemon or orange flavors, playing with toys that were cold and smooth (magnetic balls), listening to country music, and rubbing a soft baby blanket.

Step 4: Teach Coping Skills

Breathing retraining was introduced and Mary responded favorably. She immediately felt better after practicing. In addition, a list of coping statements was created to help Mary stay focused on the treatment and encourage her to remain in the uncomfortable situation without escape or avoidance. These statements included:

"I have a sensitive nervous system."

"There is no emergency."

"Even though I don't care for a feeling, I can work with my new skills and stay in the situation."

"I can deal with yucky smells and yucky feelings."

"I can practice deep breathing and wash my hands after touching the dog to get the wet slobber off."

"I can handle this."

Step 5: Incorporate Counterconditioning

Mary and her therapist discussed making a fun experience out of encounters with dogs. First, she and her mother searched the Internet for pictures of the cutest dogs in the world. They identified the 10 cutest dogs (to Mary) and looked up breeders in the area. Eventually, she wanted to visit these breeders to see if the dogs were as cute in person as in the pictures. Next, Mary thought it might be fun to go to the house of a family friend who has a very well-trained dog and have the dog follow commands such as "sit," "shake," or "roll over." Mary was intrigued with the idea that the dog would listen to her. Her therapist also suggested that when she greets a dog, she should always put her hand out to allow the dog to smell her and possibly lick her hand. In this way, she is controlling where and when the dog licks and smells and possibly avoid later smelling and licking from the dog. Finally, Mary thought it might be fun to attend a dog training class to watch how the dogs are trained and see how commands are taught to the animals.

Step 6: Institute a Reward System

Mary and her parents discussed using a reward system. They agreed that Mary would earn points each time she practiced her coping skills, used sensory interventions, and worked with the exposure hierarchy. Mary would cash in her points each day to receive different art supplies. Because Mary loved markers, pastels, paints, sketch pads, and many types of craft activities, Mary's parents purchased the art supplies before Mary started working on her hierarchy so that she could immediately earn a reward as soon as she began working with her new therapeutic skills.

Step 7: Implement a Comprehensive Treatment Plan

Mary began her treatment by practicing breathing retraining in the morning before school and at night before bed. Mary also read her coping statements at the same time. Mary discovered some citrus oils at a health food store that she rubbed under her nose to create pleasant aromas all day long. Mary started to suck on hard candy before taking a bath and listened to country music for 15 minutes each evening while playing with her blanket and magnetic balls. These activities all seem to help Mary feel better in general. Mary was particularly thrilled that while she was beginning to feel more comfortable, she was also earning some appealing art supplies.

At session four, Mary and her therapist walked to a nearby dog park and viewed the dogs from outside the fence. They rated the cuteness or desirability of each dog that she saw. Before leaving the office, she put the citrus oil under her nose, put in her earbuds to listen to music, and carried her magnetic stones with her. During this session, Mary was able to touch a dog and allow it to lick her hand. She was very uncomfortable during the exposure but was thrilled with her progress in just 1 hour. She agreed to practice several times before the next session.

At the next session, Mary's therapist brought her very calm golden retriever, Rex, and had Rex sit in on the session on a leash, on the floor near the therapist. Mary did eventually allow Rex to lick her hand and she petted Rex, but Mary did not want Rex to be let off his leash or to approach her. By session eight, Mary and Rex had played together with Rex off his leash, she had experimented with Rex licking different parts of her body, and she had even given Rex a hairdo by brushing his long golden fur.

As Mary worked on her hierarchy, her confidence grew. Using her sensory interventions and coping skills, she was able to practice exposures of increasing difficulty repeatedly until she had completed her hierarchy. Her parents were positive and encouraging and praised her hard work, which felt really good to her. Three months after the start of therapy, Mary and her therapist terminated treatment.

SPECIFIC PHOBIA

Ian was a happy 12-year-old when he entered middle school. He was a good student, had friends, and played soccer and basketball. During the first few weeks of middle school there was a fire drill. All of the kids lined up and exited the school. Ian was completely startled by the drill. The sound was so much louder than the alarm at his elementary school. When Ian returned to the classroom he could not concentrate. He felt his heart racing and was preoccupied with the thought that there might be another alarm. He told his teacher that he did not feel well, went to the nurse's office, and was able to go home. Since that day, Ian has been having a great deal of difficulty going to school and staying focused. While he was a B student in elementary school, Ian has barely been able to maintain a D average due to his fear of the fire alarm. As a result of the decline in his grades and functioning, Ian's parents sought professional help.

Step 1: Make the Diagnosis and Provide Education

The therapist first met with Ian's parents to learn more about Ian's developmental history and the history of his presenting phobia. Ian's parents reported that prior to the fire alarm in middle school, he had a generally uneventful time in elementary school. They observed that when Ian was very young, he would cover his ears when flushing the toilet and frequently asked his parents not to yell when they were speaking in what they thought were normal voices. As Ian grew older, his parents noted that he would ask his friends to be quiet when they played with him, and he could not sleep with the normal sounds around the house at night and required a white noise machine in his room to fall asleep. Because Ian was able to maintain his friendships and, with the addition of the noise machine, was able to fall asleep, Ian's parents thought these were just quirks of his. However, they became quite concerned when he exhibited such an overreaction to the fire drill at school.

The therapist spoke to Ian about his experience with sounds while growing up. Ian said that certain sounds felt overwhelming to him. His ears would hurt, his heart would race, and he felt really uncomfortable, like he had to run away when he heard certain sounds. He was particularly vulnerable to this anxious reaction when the sound was unexpected or unpredictable. Thus, the fire drill was the worst. Ian lived in constant fear at school because he was preoccupied with the anticipation of the noise of the drill.

Ian was so upset that he started to actively avoid school for fear that an alarm might go off. When he did attend school, Ian was unable to concentrate on his schoolwork due to his preoccupation with the possibility of an alarm. Based on parent report, Ian's self-report, and the answers to the Sensory Checklist found in Chapter 3, Ian's therapist determined that Ian's anxiety about alarms was driven by sensory sensitivities and a overreactivity to sound. The therapist explained sensory dysregulation to Ian and his parents and described how certain sounds feel uncomfortable and overwhelming to Ian, which leads him to feel anxious and feel like he must flee from the situation. This feeling leads to active avoidance, which reinforces the fear and discomfort.

Step 2: Create an Exposure Hierarchy

Ian's therapist explained the treatment to him. Ian was very interested from the start. He was eager to get back to school and conquer his fear of alarms. He was sick of feeling uncomfortable and left out. Ian and his therapist discussed the types of sounds that really bothered him, and together they created a hierarchy:

1. Look at a picture of an alarm.
2. Listen to a very soft (barely audible) alarm sound (found on the Internet).
3. Listen to the alarm sound at progressively higher volumes.
4. (Have parents go to the school and record the sound of the actual alarm.) Listen to the school alarm softly.

5. Listen to the sound of the school alarm at progressively higher volumes.

6. Listen to the recording of the school alarm in an empty school building on a weekend or late in the day on a week-day.

7. Do homework at school (weekend or late in the day) and have a parent play the alarm but not inform Ian as to when it will sound (element of surprise).

8. Have the school allow Ian to be at school on a Saturday, and sound the alarm while he is studying.

9. Attend school with a warning that the alarm will sound at a specific time.

10. Experience the alarm unexpectedly while he is at school.

Step 3: Teach Sensory Interventions

Ian and his therapist explored some different sensory experiences that he might find soothing. The sensory interventions that Ian found calming included chewing sour gum (apple, grape, or cherry), playing with a textured ball (a koosh-type ball or a goo-filled ball felt the best), playing with kinetic sand, wearing a snug knit cap, and listening to music. Ian's parents worked with him to collect these items so that he would have easy access when he needed to use them.

Step 4: Teach Coping Skills

Ian was taught deep breathing as a form of relaxation training. This made sense to him because of his years on sports teams. Deep breathing and breath control were important in basketball, and his coach had been working with the whole team on this. Ian was really excited to use this skill while at school, at home, and on the basketball court.

Ian and his therapist also created a list of coping statements that encouraged him to stay in the situation and resist the urge to flee:

"I have a sensitive nervous system."

"My nervous system sometimes sends me error messages just like my computer does."

"Alarms are loud, but I can manage them."

"I will use my deep breathing and sensory interventions to help me cope."

"I do not have to flee. I can stay here and use my skills."

Ian started to read his coping statements every morning before school and at night before bed. In addition to using coping statements, his therapist taught him to time the alarm. He would practice using a stopwatch or using the second hand on his watch each time the alarm sounded. This allowed him to use timing as a distraction from the alarm itself. Eventually he learned to count in his head (e.g., one-one-thousand, two-one-thousand, three-one-thousand). Ian liked using this strategy because it gave him something to do in his head, which kept his focus away from anticipating the next alarm.

Step 5: Incorporate Counterconditioning

Ian's therapist talked to Ian about counterconditioning. He explained that including a fun activity during a challenging one can alter the experience by providing a positive distraction while staying in a challenging situation. Ian and his therapist talked about looking for something specific once the alarm sounded to distract him from the sound, such as noticing who was the first person to walk out of the classroom, counting the number of people who wore socks, or seeing how many people were jumping up and down due to cool weather. Ian liked the idea of looking for people wearing socks and decided to count them the first time there was a fire drill.

Step 6: Institute a Reward System

The therapist spoke with Ian and his parents about using a reward system. Ian really loved to make models of cars, boats, and airplanes.

Ian and his parents decided that he could earn pieces of a model each day. For an inexpensive model, he could earn the pieces for the entire model by the end of the week. A larger, more intricate model could be earned over the course of 2 to 3 weeks. Ian loved this idea and was willing to work on his hierarchy to earn the reward.

Step 7: Implement a Comprehensive Treatment Plan

Ian began practicing deep breathing right away. He practiced at night before he fell asleep and in the morning before going to school. Reading coping statements was quickly added. He would read them immediately before practicing his breathing. Ian began to earn points for practice and was excited to earn a model airplane at the end of the first week. Ian noticed that he was a bit more comfortable and started to focus on his breathing and coping statements, rather than being preoccupied by thinking about when the alarm might sound.

Ian's mother got permission for Ian to wear a knit cap and chew gum in school. Ian found a pencil with a koosh ball topper and was able to use it in all of his classes. He found that being able to use these techniques in school made him feel more comfortable and confident.

Ian was able to start at level 3 of the hierarchy (listening to progressively louder alarm sounds at home) and was up to level 6 by the end of the week. Ian's parents were thrilled and had to scramble to make sure they were prepared for his next step in therapy. His parents needed to record the school fire alarm and secure permission to be in the school building on a weekend and listen to the fire alarm. It was very important that Ian's parents prepare ahead of time in order to be able to support Ian's growing momentum. He worked quickly up the hierarchy, listening to alarm sounds while practicing deep breathing, reciting his coping statements, counting the length of the alarm, and using his sensory interventions. By the end of the second week, Ian was practicing listening to the fire alarm at school on the weekend.

Once the treatment was in place and Ian began to practice his relaxation skills, coping skills, and sensory interventions, Ian's confidence soared. He and his parents were surprised at how quickly

Ian was able to move through his hierarchy and manage his discomfort to return to school daily. Before the end of the month, Ian was able to successfully tolerate the fire alarm sounding, unexpectedly, while he was at school.

ATTENTION-DEFICIT/
HYPERACTIVITY DISORDER

Audrey is a 7-year-old second grader. She was full of energy and in constant motion at home. She was bright, inquisitive, and highly verbal. It was hard for her to wait her turn and she frequently blurted things out at school. Audrey's teacher notified her parents about behaviors that concerned her. The teacher observed that Audrey frequently got into fights when lining up with the class to leave the classroom. Audrey regularly tattled on kids who were not following the rules. She would regularly blurt out questions without raising her hand and frequently ask the teacher to repeat the directions that had just been given. Audrey would squirm in her seat, and the constant movement and blurting out would disturb the other children. When corrected, which the teacher often did, Audrey would dissolve into tears. Audrey spent a lot of time out of the classroom in trouble or upset, talking with the nurse, guidance counselor, or an administrator. Audrey's teacher asked them if she could be evaluated for ADHD. As a result, her parents decided to seek professional help.

Step 1: Make the Diagnosis and Provide Education

Audrey's parents reported to the therapist what the teacher had observed. They added that Audrey had always been a high-energy child. She achieved her developmental milestones such as walking and talking earlier than expected. She was naturally inquisitive and very verbal. She has never been satisfied with simple explanations and always sought more information. Audrey's mom described her as a whirling dervish because she was in constant motion and was unable to sit still for even a short period of time. She liked to stand and bounce as she talked. When she wasn't talking and bouncing, Audrey would be running around, spinning, jumping, touching, and picking up objects. When Audrey was a toddler, her parents were exhausted trying to keep up with her. They channeled her high energy into many playdates, gymnastics, and swim classes to wear her out. Audrey also has never been a good sleeper: she was hard to settle down and frequently tossed and turned for several hours before falling asleep. In the morning, she was very difficult to wake and frequently resisted getting out of bed and getting ready for school.

Audrey did very well in preschool and early elementary school. She was a quick learner and picked up concepts before the other children. Her preschool, kindergarten, and first-grade teachers told her parents that she was the class helper, and Audrey loved that role. When Audrey finished her work, she was able to help the teacher by passing out supplies or putting away crayons, after which she could sit in the teacher's rocking chair and read. Audrey loved the movement while reading, and she really enjoyed these times. Sometimes her teachers would allow her to do jumping jacks before sitting down. Her parents said that her previous teachers noticed Audrey's high energy and tendency to cry easily, but it never seemed to pose a problem. Her parents wondered if Audrey really did have ADHD or if maybe her second-grade teacher did not understand Audrey the way her other teachers had.

The therapist gathered information from the Child Behavior Checklist (Auchenbach, 1991) and other questionnaires for parents and teachers. The teacher also requested that Audrey have some educational testing done at school because she was concerned that Audrey's behavior was beginning to affect her academic performance.

The results of all of the testing were inconclusive. Audrey had some behavioral symptoms of ADHD, but her cognitive processing and working memory were excellent; thus a diagnosis was not made, but also could not be ruled out. Audrey's therapist presented a picture of a child who had some underresponsiveness to sensory input and had some overresponsiveness to perceived criticism. She seemed to require a great deal of movement and stimulation in order to feel settled. Audrey's testing showed that she had a high need to please others and perfectionistic strivings. As a result, she reacted powerfully to correction, feeling sad and shameful about her behavior. Her therapist explained that Audrey's sensory system was dysregulated, underreacting to certain sensory stimuli and overreacting to hearing what she perceived as criticism about her character. Therapy could help her balance her reactions, feel more comfortable physically, and learn to recognize and regulate her dysregulated nervous system. Once this had been accomplished, it would be easier to determine if ADHD was also a contributing factor.

Step 2: Create an Exposure Hierarchy

Audrey and her therapist talked about the types of situations that might get her upset or in trouble at school. Using this information, they were able to create a hierarchy of exposure experiences. Audrey's hierarchy looked like this:

1. Raise her hand before she speaks up in class.
2. Wait in line quietly without telling the teacher about what other children are doing.
3. Accept correction of her behavior gracefully.
4. Limit the number of her questions.
5. Stand still while talking.
6. Sit in her seat in the classroom, looking at the teacher or the chalkboard/screen.

Each of these tasks seemed equally challenging for Audrey, so she did not rank them in ascending order. She felt that she could work on all of these behaviors, but wanted to start one at a time. The therapist agreed, as she tends toward perfectionism, to start slow to ensure some initial success and not put her in a situation where she would experience self-criticism.

Step 3: Teach Sensory Interventions

Audrey's therapist applauded her enthusiasm for working on these behaviors and suggested that there were some skills that might help her be more successful as she tried to improve her behavior. This really appealed to Audrey, and she was eager to learn.

The therapist reminded Audrey that her body liked a lot of movement to settle down. Recess and after school-activities were excellent times to achieve this goal. During school, however, Audrey should concentrate on focusing on smaller movements and teach her body to be interested and satisfied with different types of sensory input. These sensory interventions would also help Audrey soothe herself.

Audrey and her therapist made two lists of sensory interventions, one appropriate for use in school and one for use outside of school. The in-school list of sensory interventions included: wearing a stretchy beaded bracelet and playing with the beads, using pen and pencil toppers that had some tactile appeal, playing discreetly with small koosh balls, animal-shaped erasers or fluffy puff balls, using pen and pencil grippers with different types of textures, and using putty erasers. Audrey could also chew strong-flavored gum or suck on strong-flavored mints (peppermint or green apple).

Outside of school Audrey's intervention list included sit on a large ball or rocking chair while reading or doing homework, use pen or pencil toppers and grippers while writing, suck on extremely sour candy, play with Silly Putty, listen to music (classical or music without lyrics), run up and down the stairs 10 times before settling down to do homework, do 20 jumping jacks every 30 minutes during homework, and sit on a wiggle cushion while reading or doing homework.

These sensory interventions, practiced both at home and at school, would help Audrey function more comfortably in both environments. Audrey's mother needed to contact the school, explain the reasoning behind using the interventions in the classroom, and negotiate which interventions Audrey could utilize while sitting at her desk.

Step 4: Teach Coping Skills

Breathing retraining and progressing muscle relaxation were introduced to Audrey. These skills provided a different way for her body to gain some sensory input and to settle down without requiring excessive movement. She practiced these skills every night before bed. Over time, she learned to settle herself to sleep in less than 30 minutes, which allowed her 30–90 minutes of additional sleep per night.

Audrey and her therapist created a list of coping statements to help Audrey focus on her skills.

"Sometimes my behavior is more active, but I am a good person."

"I have a sensitive nervous system."

"My body likes to move a lot, but I can't jump around in every situation."

"My body will learn to like the sensory toys."

"I am not perfect, nobody is."

"When my teacher corrects me, she is trying to help."

"It's OK to have a lot of energy, I can learn to manage it."

"The teacher is in charge of the class, I don't have tell her about the other children."

"Sometimes kids will not follow the rules. Nobody is perfect."

"I can handle it when the exact rules are not followed."

Audrey practiced her breathing skills each evening before bed and in the morning before school. She also read her coping statements at the same time.

Step 5: Incorporate Counterconditioning

Audrey was fully engaged in the treatment process and the therapist chose not to include counterconditioning into her treatment plan at this time.

Step 6: Institute a Reward System

Audrey's teacher made a behavioral chart that was kept private from the class. They would briefly discuss the chart both after lunch and at the end of the day. On the chart were items for which she could earn points: raising her hand before talking, using her sensory toys discreetly in class, keeping her hands to herself and her body reasonably still. Each day Audrey would see her success in each area and, because the chart was checked at a midway point, she could correct behaviors that needed work.

Audrey and her parents discussed the types of rewards that Audrey would like to receive while working on managing these behaviors. Audrey had attended a party recently and really loved all of the small items she received in her goody bag. Audrey thought she might like to earn a goody bag item each day. Her parents thought that this was a great idea. In order to earn a reward, Audrey needed to earn more than half of the points possible for each day. If Audrey earned all of the possible points on any given day, she would receive two toys. Her parents ordered dozens of small toys from an online store. In addition, her parents kept a chart at home for her school successes. Each day when the report came home, they would track her successes on a sticker chart, so that she could see her progress.

This reward system was a critical piece of Audrey's treatment. She had been receiving a great deal of negative feedback in school and was feeling sad and defeated. Being able to receive rewards and see her progress significantly improved her mood and improved her motivation to work on behavior change.

Step 7: Implement a Comprehensive Treatment Plan

Audrey first started to practice her coping skills at home. She immediately received rewards for her efforts, and her parents saw an improvement in her behavior right away. Using the daily feedback from the teacher, a baseline for her behavior was established. Audrey's pretreatment behavior included bothering the children sitting close to her by her constant movement, crying at least once each day, tattling on others, and calling out without raising her hand 10–12 times a day. After one week of practice at home, Audrey began to use her sensory interventions and her new coping skills at school as well. Audrey's behavior began to improve quickly, as evidenced in her daily teacher reports—crying only once a week rather than once a day, sitting reasonably still and not bothering children seated close to her, tattling once every three to four days, and raising her hand and waiting her turn to speak without blurting out answers. Some days were better than others. Both Audrey's parents and her teacher concentrated on noticing the positive, not focusing on the negative. This strategy was particularly helpful for Audrey because she was so sensitive to criticism. Both her parents and teacher observed that simply commenting on the positive and ignoring the negative had a much more positive impact on her behavior than when they commented on the negative.

Audrey made great progress at home and at school. By the end of the school year, Audrey had vastly reduced her crying (largely due to the reduction in negative comments), was able to stand in line without tattling on her friends, and was able to sit at her desk without squirming or bothering her neighbors. These improvements were recognized by the teacher, the school counselor, and the school nurse. In addition, her peer relationships improved dramatically. She still sometimes called out in class a bit, bounced occasionally while she stood, and asked more questions than the other children, but overall she was a happier and more highly functioning child.

OPPOSITIONAL DEFIANT DISORDER

Travis is an 11-year-old boy who presented for treatment with a previous diagnosis of ODD, OCD, Tourette syndrome, and ADHD. He had been evaluated by a psychologist and was referred for behavioral treatment of ODD and anxiety. His mother described him as a sweet child who, over the past 5 years, had decided to systematically refuse to do anything that he was asked to do. He refused to wear new clothes, go to a friend's house, eat new foods, help out around the house, and even to touch objects that he did not want to touch.

Step 1: Make the Diagnosis and Provide Education

Travis was clear that the origin of his discomfort was a dislike for stickiness. It started with touching stickers when he was younger and not liking the way they felt on his fingers. Later he began to avoid things that potentially could be sticky, like new clothes or objects such as trash. He had the experience of wearing a shirt that had a sticker on it previously and still had sticky residue on it. He flat-out refused to ever again wear new clothes, even if they had been washed prior to wearing. This generalized to new shoes and new backpacks for school. When pushed to do something he did not want to do or when he was feeling overwhelmed, he would grimace and make vocal noises that seemed inconsistent with the environment, which is how he got the Tourette syndrome diagnosis. At school he would repeatedly touch or come close to touching other children, even after being told, "Stop it." His parents became very worried about his ability to function in the world, despite his superior IQ.

After further evaluation, including evaluation of the sensory system, his therapist changed the working diagnoses to ADHD (which was very evident in his educational testing) and sensory dysregulation with oppositional and anxious features.

Many sessions were spent initially with both Travis and his family to explain the sensory nervous system and how it is greatly impacting Travis's functioning. His sensitivity to sticky tactile sensations caused initial discomfort, which over time has turned into anxiety, avoidance, and oppositional behavior. It is the anxious avoidance that looks like ODD and OCD. Travis was very slow to warm up to the therapist, who had to be very careful not to push too hard, while laying the foundation to eventually gain his acceptance of the treatment goals. He was able to identify that his avoidance was causing a problem for him but was not at all sure that he wanted to do anything about it. Building rapport and trust was a process that in this case took six sessions to accomplish. His therapist got to witness his noise making and his avoidant behavior (walking out), which were explained to him as his nervous system's way of soothing itself and blocking out things that were upsetting to him. Simply normalizing this behavior helped him to feel less weird and more like a normal kid. Finally, at the seventh session, he and his therapist were able to make a plan for moving forward.

Step 2: Create an Exposure Hierarchy

Travis and his therapist created an exposure hierarchy that he was able to accept and agree upon:

1. Look at stickers without touching them.
2. Touch the front side of a sticker.

3. Touch a new T-shirt that he and his mom inspected for stickers.

4. Wear a T-shirt that had no stickers on it to begin with.

5. Wear a T-shirt that had a sticker on it but had been washed.

6. Wear a new T-shirt that he was not sure had ever had a sticker on it.

7. Touch new objects (in session at first) that might feel sticky.

8. Touch putty, slime, goo, and other sticky substances (first in session, then at home).

9. Apply glue to his fingers and allow it to feel sticky.

10. Go to new places (the mall, an amusement park, a carnival) that might have stickiness and touch things accordingly.

Both Travis and his parents agreed that these exposures would take time, and everyone agreed to be patient during the process. Everyone agreed that Travis would be able to say "Too much" and set limits if he felt too pressured. Having this control over the exposures was the only way to get him to buy in to the process. Travis's avoidance and oppositional behavior were dealt with by giving him some control over the situation, which allowed him to face situations that were previously avoided.

Step 3: Teach Sensory Intervention

Before ever beginning the exposure process, Travis had to work on sensory soothing. Parts of the first six sessions were spent exploring what sensations were pleasing to him and how to incorporate these into his life. Because he was hesitant to touch new objects out of concern for stickiness, tactile soothing was left until the end. His therapist started with auditory sensations. Travis clearly used his voice and noise to soothe himself, so his therapist started here. They learned that he really loved hard rock music, and that listening to this was calming to him. Unfortunately, listening to hard rock music was not at all soothing to his parents. He was allowed and encouraged to listen to his music while getting dressed in the morning, but he was encouraged to use his headphones while doing homework and during the car ride to school so as not to disturb others in the same environment. His parents had been discouraging this type of music because they do not like it. When they learned that this is a way for him to self-soothe, they were more accepting.

Interestingly, Travis had a very low sensitivity for smell. He was able to go into very smelly places and not react at all. This had always puzzled his parents because of his strange reactions to other situations. When experimenting with the sense of smell, Travis and his therapist learned that he really likes the smell of pungent eucalyptus. His mother bought him a bottle of eucalyptus essential oil. He would put some oil on a napkin and keep it in his pocket. He would smell it during the day when he felt upset or frustrated with something. He liked the way it gave him a sense of control over the way he felt and responded favorably to using it.

Chewing gum served as a distraction from his other senses, and he liked being allowed to chew gum more regularly. His parents consulted with his school, and he was granted permission to chew gum in class. He was thrilled with this privilege and did not flaunt it in front of his peers.

Finally, Travis and his therapist learned that he really liked to touch soft things, like a chenille blanket. He also preferred smooth objects to rough ones, so some smooth stones were located and he carried them with him at all times. After weeks of practicing with these sensory interventions, he was a much calmer and more settled child. His parents reported that he seemed settled internally, was less argumentative, and that the noise making and grimacing had diminished greatly. This, coupled with his parents not pushing him, allowed the entire family to get along better and have more positive interactions overall.

Step 4: Teach Coping Skills

During the first weeks of active treatment, Travis was taught deep breathing techniques and visualization. In each session he and his therapist would practice doing a deep relaxation sequence with a visualization of him lying on a raft in a pool on a warm, sunny day, floating in peace. He liked practicing this visualization and made a recording of it in session so he could practice it at home. After weeks of practice, Travis reported that he was able to just close his eyes and imagine himself floating and could re-create this relaxing feeling within himself.

Step 5: Incorporate Counterconditioning

Travis had an affinity for games, particularly video games where he could earn points. He and his therapist employed a game approach to the hierarchy. Travis would pretend he was a Pac man chasing a sticky ghost. When he encountered a sticky item, Travis would envelop it, holding it close to his skin and clothing. This behavior simulated Pac man eating the ghosts. Using Pac man as a model encouraged Travis to truly engage with the sticky item rather than to simply timidly touch it. In addition, he could earn lots of points for his continued brave efforts. To tally the points, he would multiply the number of exposures by the level of exposures each day (e.g., if he did three level 1's, he would get 3 points, while if he did two level 8's, he would get 16 points). Travis learned quickly that he liked to win the higher points and pushed himself to try harder exposures. Again, this was important because it was his idea, and he controlled the pace and the level of exposure. His parents realized that their pushing was a large part of his oppositional behavior. When they allowed him to have some control over his environment, he stepped up more quickly.

Step 6: Institute a Reward System

Travis's parents used the point system to help him get rewards. He wanted to earn iTunes gift cards to download more hard rock music and game playing time. They worked out a system to make clear how he could earn these two things. He was thrilled to be able to control his music library as well as his ability to play his favorite video games.

Step 7: Implement a Comprehensive Treatment Plan

For Travis, as for many children who have issues with sensory dysregulation, most of the work took place prior to any exposures even occurring. He was only able to do the exposure work after he had practiced skill building and sensory soothing. At the first exposure session, he and his therapist listened to his favorite heavy metal band while throwing a sticky splat ball against the window. They discovered that he was able to jump up the hierarchy to a higher level when music was incorporated. This made some of the lower exposures more approachable. Once he started the exposure work, he was able to work through his hierarchy over the next 12 weeks and was able to reach his goal of going places and touching things that were unfamiliar. Eventually, Travis began to increase his confidence and expertly manage his discomfort with stickiness, and his defiance eventually subsided.

COMPULSIVE SKIN PICKING

Molly is a 13-year-old eighth grader. She presented for treatment of skin picking disorder, with symptoms that had waxed and waned since her parents could remember but had worsened over the past year. Last summer, Molly spent a week at the beach with family friends and got lots of mosquito bites. She scratched them until they bled and formed scabs, then she picked off the scabs. When she returned home after a week, her arms and legs were completely covered in scabs and open, bleeding sores. In addition, in the past 6 months she had started to have acne breakouts on her face, which also triggered her to pick. Her parents had tried reminding her to stop picking, which only made her more frustrated. Molly's parents were concerned that she would develop infections or permanent scarring on her body.

Step 1: Make the Diagnosis and Provide Education

During the initial intake it became obvious that Molly had always been very sensory focused. Her parents described her early on as a thumb sucker who needed to suck and rub her blanket at all times. As a young child she disliked loud noise, could not tolerate certain smells, bit her fingernails, and had a favorite stuffed animal that she rubbed until it no longer had fur. Molly's parents were very receptive to the idea that her issues had a sensory origin, and her mom even acknowledged that she was very much the same way as a child and engaged in hair pulling (also a sensory-based behavior) for 10 years of her life.

Step 2: Create an Exposure Hierarchy

When creating a treatment plan for compulsive skin picking and hair pulling, exposure may be part of the treatment package, but additional techniques also should be incorporated that identify and address various internal and external triggers. Sensory experiences are classified as internal triggers. For example, Molly described her desire to feel smooth skin and how the rough image or feel of a scab or bump caused her to experience discomfort, as if her skin needed to be smoothed out or fixed. Feelings, thoughts, and beliefs are examples of other internal triggers, while places, activities, and objects (mirrors, razors, needles) are examples of common external triggers. In order for persons to change skin-picking or hair-pulling behavior, they must be able to either learn to tolerate the uncomfortable trigger and not respond to it by picking or pulling, or to reduce sensory-seeking aspects of pulling/picking (e.g., watching all of the excoriate come out of a pimple and feeling gratified by this process).

For Molly, the uncomfortable sensory experiences were visual (noticing a bump, scab, or blemish) and tactile (feeling a scab, pimple, bump, raised area, or rough patch). She would scan her body, consciously and unconsciously, for anything that looked or felt raised, rough, or red. Initially, she was not able to resist picking when something was identified, even for a short period of time. Her exposure hierarchy looked like this:

1. Allow a scab to heal and form new skin after identifying it visually.
2. Allow a scab to heal and form new skin after identifying it through touch.
3. Allow a pimple to heal without picking at it after identifying it visually.
4. Allow a pimple to heal without picking at it after identifying it through touch.

These four exposure activities required a great deal of support and alteration of the environment for her to be successful.

Step 3: Teach Sensory Intervention

Sensory interventions for Molly were introduced at the onset of treatment. Because she liked the smooth feeling of skin, her therapist started with objects that felt smooth. Molly identified that magnetic balls, smooth stones, and soft blankets were all appealing to her. Because much of her picking took place while she was in bed at night, her mom bought her some satin pajamas (which allowed her to feel smooth fabric against her skin) and satin gloves (which prevented her from being able to feel irregularities on her skin). When she was away from home, she wore bracelets with large, smooth stones so that she could feel the smooth sensation. Another pleasing sensory sensation was Thinking Putty, which Molly discovered had a very smooth feel and did not leave any residue on her hands after she played with it. These sensory objects were strategically placed in environments where Molly typically picked her skin. She practiced using them in these environments for several weeks until the strategy use became part of her new routine.

Step 4: Teach Coping Skills

Coping strategies for Molly included covering her scabs with thin blister bandages that were water resistant. Molly found that the thin bandages created a visual and tactile barrier that took away the rough, bumpy look and feel so that she was able to forget about the area while the bandages were on. Because these bandages are water resistant, they tend to stay on for several days at a time. Other coping skills included limiting her time in the bathroom (where there are bright lights, mirrors, and a tendency to be unclothed). She used a kitchen timer when she went into the bathroom to get ready in the morning and in the evening before bedtime. Because acne breakouts were a trigger for Molly, her mother took her to a dermatologist to get treatment for her pimples. She was prescribed some facial wash and cream to reduce the breakouts that were triggering her face picking.

Step 5: Incorporate Counterconditioning

There was no counterconditioning for this treatment. Molly was able to fully participate and engage in treatment with the use a reward system and did not require this intervention.

Step 6: Institute a Reward System

Molly was able to receive rewards for using her various strategies both at home and at school. When her parents or teachers observed her using a strategy, she would receive a check mark. At the end of the day, Molly would count up all of the check marks and write down a total for the day on her chart. Each day she would try to earn more check marks than the previous day. If she earned less than the previous day, she would simply have less to earn the next day to beat the day before. Molly and her parents felt like this was a very straightforward and simple way to acknowledge the positive use of interventions and not focus on the negative behavior of picking. After five daily successes, Molly could earn a $10 gift card to her favorite store. She wanted to save up her gift cards to purchase items of greater value over time. Molly's parents were instructed to refrain from any nagging behavior, to give positive verbal reinforcement for using strategies, and to focus on other important things about Molly, like her ability to play soccer and her knack for geography. They shifted their attention from skin picking to positive aspects of Molly's life.

Step 7: Implement a Comprehensive Treatment Plan

Molly started treatment by using her sensory interventions and incorporating her coping skills. Her parents shifted to a more positive focus and use of the reward system. With all of these pieces in place, she was ready to begin exposure work. Her parents noticed that through these interventions alone, her picking had decreased dramatically, though they hadn't even talked about reducing the behavior. Molly was surprised that improvement could happen by using sensory interventions and coping skills.

The first exposure took place in session with her parents present. First she took out her sensory soothing interventions and started playing with them. She was then asked to find a spot on her body that felt rough or that she might want to pick. Molly found a scab that she had recently created through picking. She rated her desire to pick this scab as a 7 on a scale of 1–10. At his point her therapist started to time the exposure with a stopwatch. Molly was instructed to focus on the rough spot. Molly described her urge to pick to the therapist by talking about where in her body she felt the urge to pick (in her fingers), what emotions she experienced while having an urge (frustration), and any thoughts that emerged while sitting with the urge (I need to remove this now). Molly's therapist timed this exchange and asked her to signal when her urge to pick diminished. Molly was surprised to learn that her urge started to decline after only 90 seconds. This information was extremely helpful. However, Molly did identify that she was highly uncomfortable during those 90 seconds. To address her sensory sensations in her fingers, she was instructed to play with various sensory items, changing them frequently as she tired of them. To address her frustration, she was asked to take deep breaths and imagine breathing out her frustration. To address her automatic thought "I need to remove this now," she was asked to come up with several coping statements or challenge statements. Molly came up with several:

"If I do not remove this now, it will heal."
"This feeling will pass and I will be OK."

During the first exposure her therapist also introduced some sensory interventions that provided sensory input to other parts of her body. She tried a head massager that made Molly's scalp tingle. Molly found this sensation to be stimulating and almost like a tickle. Although Molly's urge to pick began to diminish after 90 seconds, it took the entire exposure, which lasted just under 5 minutes, for Molly to rate the strength of her urge at a 1. She learned that she was able to experience an urge to pick without needing act on it when she used her strategies. Her parents were instructed to follow the same procedures to help Molly engage in active practice on a daily basis.

   In the first week of active treatment, Molly discovered that when she used sensory interventions prior to feeling a desire to pick her skin, she often felt no urge at all. This was very surprising and relieving to her. She identified vulnerable environments where she might otherwise pick and began to use multiple strategies (cognitive coping, relaxation techniques, sensory interventions) upon entering the specific room or place. With the use of environmental modifications and active practice, including sensory interventions, coping skills, and rewards, Molly was able to allow her wounds to heal. She eventually stopped picking to a noticeable degree altogether.

CONCLUSION

Sensory dysregulation is a transdiagnostic issue that can affect individuals across the lifespan. Many times it occurs alongside, or can mimic, a psychological disorder. This chapter reviewed the treatment of children with a variety of psychological disorders, explaining how it can be modified to address specific symptoms of sensory dysregulation in the context of CBT. This modified treatment, using the formula Exposure + Sensory Intervention + Coping Skills + Counterconditioning = Tolerance for the sensory stimulus, yields effective, positive behavior change when other treatments have not been successful. The next chapter presents common challenges to treatment, as well as discusses how to navigate treatment successfully.

CHAPTER 9

Troubleshooting
in Therapy

Therapy can be complicated when providing treatment for a child who has a dysregulated nervous system. This chapter addresses some common "red flags" that may indicate the need to evaluate and address sensory issues, as well as common complicating factors that need troubleshooting.

CLUES FOR WHEN TO EVALUATE
FOR SENSORY DYSREGULATION

Probably one of the more obvious situations that may cause a therapist to reevaluate treatment is when the patient and family are actively participating in treatment and the therapy is not yielding the results that should be expected. This red flag indicates the need for an evaluation for other possible underlying factors, including sensory dysregulation. When the etiology of a symptom is sensory, rather than anxiety related, a child will not respond to exposure therapy in typical ways, meaning that she does not experience habituation to the trigger stimulus because the driving force is not anxiety. Ideally, this need to address the sensory system would be identified early on or at the onset of treatment so that frustration and a lack of progress can be avoided, but this is not always possible, that is, the sensory dysregulation gets missed. When treatment is not progressing as would be expected despite client participation, consider evaluation of the sensory system.

Another red flag for sensory dysregulation is the presence of multiple diagnoses, none of which completely explains the child's behavior. In cases such as these, often it is the dysregulated nervous system that is the source of the symptomatology, not the ADHD, OCD, generalized anxiety disorder, ODD, phobia, and so forth. A dysregulated nervous system can look like so many different psychological disorders, and depending on what type of professional children have seen in the past, they often come to therapy with between four and six diagnoses already. Understanding the true nature of the behavior and the driving forces behind it can really help therapy progress in a meaningful manner. Viewing the dysregulated nervous system as the genesis of multiple diagnoses provides a more cohesive understanding of the child's varied symptoms. The dysregulated nervous system can be compared to the trunk of a tree, from which multiple branches (the diagnoses) extend. This is not to say that numerous psychological disorders cannot exist simultaneously or that the presence of multiple psychopathologies always points to sensory dysregulation, but it is certainly worth consideration when formulating a diagnostic impression and treatment plan.

Finally, it is often the case that a child has engaged in psychological testing and the results are inconclusive. Sometimes the report will reflect that there are features of or a subclinical threshold for a disorder, but the child will not actually meet criteria for the disorder. In cases such as these, there may be another driving force that needs to be evaluated. In sum, key indicators one might want to assess for sensory dysregulation are:

- The child has been in therapy previously with little positive outcome;
- Therapy is not progressing as expected despite active participation from client and family;
- The child has multiple diagnoses, none of which completely explain the behavior; and
- Psychological testing does not yield definitive results.

COMPLICATING ISSUES
THAT FREQUENTLY OCCUR

Parent–Child Interactions

As described in detail in Chapter 7, parents may unknowingly complicate the therapy process. Actions that unintentionally reinforce maladaptive behavior include accommodating the child's behavior by allowing the child to avoid situations, giving feedback that reinforces avoidant or dysfunctional behavior, supporting avoidance by performing activities for the child, and not punishing behavior that needs a consequence.

Other times, parents can be unduly harsh or critical. Sometimes parents may actually shame their child for his reactivity, failing to understand that his behavior is not simply acting out or disrespect, but the result of a neurological dysfunction.

Early in treatment, it is important to glean a full historical evaluation of how a child's behavior has been understood, managed, and responded to by the family (nuclear and extended). Once past reactions have been identified, plans for modifying these behaviors can be formulated. Providing education to parents about their child's unique nervous system is a key first step. Explain how their child's nervous system is having difficulty interpreting, integrating, or directing action accurately and/or productively, which ultimately results in observable behavioral problems. Help parents understand there is no fault or blame involved. Parents would not blame their child for having a thyroid problem any more than they should blame her for having a dysregulated nervous system. After helping parents develop compassion for their child, the next step is to redirect their behavior toward being supportive, but not accommodating.

Parents Who Are Unsupportive of Therapy

Another common issue when working with children is lack of support by a parent or other family member for the therapeutic plan or therapy in general. Many times only one parent will show up for therapy, sometimes making excuses for the other. When there is inconsistent parenting (one parent modifies behavior due to therapeutic recommendations, while the other seems unwilling to change), things can get complicated. It is usually a good idea to encourage the uninvolved parent to come in for one or more therapy sessions to help get him or her on board with treatment—or, if necessary, insist on it. Encouraging the parent to develop compassion for the child and providing education about sensory dysregulation can help. Sometimes identifying the resistant parent's own sensory sensitivities is a viable avenue. Providing an example of how uncomfortable it can be to hear the sound of nails on a chalkboard can be a good place to start. Using common unpleasant internal experiences that most of us have helps parents connect to their child's experience. Explain that it is particularly invalidating for a child when he feels misunderstood or blamed for his symptoms.

Sometimes it can be helpful to work solely with the parents for the express purpose of enlisting their participation in treatment. Devoting several sessions to exploring the parents' frustrations and anxieties may enable them to more comfortably participate in the treatment of their child. At the same time, providing parental guidance and management techniques to effectively address their child's needs can bolster parent confidence and engage them in treatment.

Parents who are reluctant about therapy might be willing to see a therapist themselves in order to help their child, even if they do not believe that they need help. That said, occasionally a parent is just too resistant to therapy to participate at all. In these unusual cases, it can help to work solely with the child and the participating parent. The reluctant parent may observe the results of the interventions and eventually open up to therapy. Either way, the child is receiving the help she needs and therapeutic progress is achieved. Sometimes engaging a grandparent, aunt, or uncle who has lots of contact with the child can be a way to garner additional family support when one parent is absent from therapy.

Parent Whose Nervous System Is at Odds with the Child's

In some cases, part of the difficulty in the home is that one of the parents also has a dysregulated nervous system, and his or her sensory system is at odds with that of the child. For example, a child may be soothed by loud rock-and-roll music or a vanilla-scented candle, and the parent may be hypersensitive to loud music or certain scents. The parent may want quiet in the house at all times or like the smell of lemon (which to the child smells like disgusting laundry detergent). In situations such as this, the therapist must first identify this incompatibility as a cause of conflict in the household, then work toward negotiating sensory experiences that the parent and child can both tolerate. In order to support therapy and reduce family conflict, the nondysregulated parent might need to take charge of some of the exposure exercises. Regardless of the approach, it is helpful to use these incompatibilities as great examples of individual differences and help both parent and child develop compassion for the other's unique nervous system and for themselves.

Multiple Children with Different Sensory Needs

Another frequent scenario is when a family has multiple children, several of whom have discrepant over- and underresponsiveness. In these types of circumstances, children can become quite upset with both parents and each other, and chaos can ensue. The best approach in families with varying sensory needs is to evaluate everyone in the family. Once the evaluation is complete, each family member should develop an understanding of "my unique nervous system." Help each of them to develop compassion, respect, and appreciation for the sensory differences among the other members of the family. For example, if Jenny knows that Mike can't stand the smell of eggs cooking (her favorite food to cook) and Jenny gets really angry when Mike chews food with his mouth open, they may have to come to some mutual agreements. Jenny might let Mike know when she is planning to cook eggs (so that he can use some sensory soothing strategies), and Mike could practice chewing his food more politely at the dinner table (which would improve his social skills as well). Learning to respect others' discrepant nervous systems and being able to talk openly about individual sensory needs is an important skill that not only normalizes sensory dysregulation, but also improves acceptance and tolerance for individual differences.

Teacher/School Resistance

Schools are typically supportive of therapeutic efforts to improve behavior and ultimately increase overall functioning for a child. Occasionally, however, a teacher or a school official will object to therapeutic recommendations or will simply not understand the goals of this type of therapy. This can be frustrating and confusing for parents. Remind parents that teachers are extremely hardworking, caring individuals who often are required to provide compassion, correction, encouragement, and individualized attention to a large number of students on a daily basis. When special adjustments or accommodation are requested, it can feel overwhelming to the teacher. Therapists (and parents) must be sensitive not only to the child, but to the teacher as well. It is useful for the therapist to talk with the teacher so that she may express her concerns about the interventions, allowing both therapist and teacher to problem-solve how to incorporate interventions into the classroom while minimizing the overall burden to the teacher. A critical point may be to help the teacher understand how therapeutic recommendations will not only benefit the child, but may also enhance overall classroom functioning.

Once a treatment plan is agreed upon, ongoing communication with the school is critical to facilitate cooperation and coordinate efforts for the benefit of the child. Many times this can be done through phone conversations or via e-mail (reports, written recommendations); however, sometimes getting permission to sit in the child's classroom or to meet with the teacher/counselor/principal in person is warranted to facilitate a coordinated treatment plan.

Occasionally a teacher or school will simply not be willing to participate in the recommendations set forth in treatment. This is unfortunate but does not have to derail treatment. If a teacher is unsupportive, help can be obtained from the school counselor, the principal, or other faculty members. This support, however, does not guarantee that the child will be allowed accommodations in the classroom or that the teacher will verbally acknowledge or reinforce positive behavior.

One such situation involved a child who worked very hard to regulate her sensory-seeking nervous system (she was constantly in motion, calling out, and disrupting the class), but despite her hard work and significant decreases in her problematic behaviors, her teacher did not acknowledge any improvement at all. Unfortunately, this teacher continued to focus on the remaining wiggling and impulsive behavior, even though there was a significant reduction in both frequency and intensity. This nonacknowledgment of improved behavior was confusing for both the child and her parents, who were perplexed by the teacher's lack of attention to treatment gains. Her parents decided to continue to work on the treatment plan despite the lack of teacher participation. They gathered information about school performance from the child and other faculty members in order to reward and reinforce the reduction of problematic behaviors in the classroom and maintained a positive attitude toward the child's improvements. This parent effort bolstered positive behavior change in a challenging, less supportive educational environment. Despite less than ideal circumstances, the child continued to make progress with the support of other faculty members and the leadership of the parents.

When the school year is close to an end, parents of children with unsupportive teachers may need to wait until the next year, with the natural change of classrooms and teachers, to implement a viable treatment plan. The hope is that the new teacher will be more open and willing to work with a targeted therapeutic program. When parents understand their child's temperament and nervous system needs, they are equipped to discuss teacher assignments with the school so that an appropriate teacher can be appointed. In other cases, requesting a teacher change is more appropriate, especially if issues are identified early in the academic year. Finally, in more extreme cases, the school itself may not be a good fit for this child if it takes a rigid stance toward behavior differences and classroom accommodation.

THE IMPORTANCE OF A TEAM APPROACH

When working with children, particularly those who have difficulty regulating their nervous systems, it is vital to take a team approach. Members of the team may include parents, grandparents (or other family members), pediatricians, psychiatrists, occupational therapists, teachers, school counselors, or athletic coaches.

Ideally, members of the team will communicate about the child's functioning in a variety of environments and be able to implement a comprehensive treatment plan that addresses physiological, emotional, educational, and neurological issues. Frequent communication about improvements in functioning, setbacks, and ongoing treatment goals is necessary so that the team is aware of how the child is functioning in a variety of contexts. Strategies for coping with difficult sensory stimuli should be shared with the team so that all involved can support and encourage the treatment process.

THE ROLE OF OCCUPATIONAL THERAPY IN TREATMENT

There is no doubt that a trained occupational therapist may be better equipped than a psychotherapist to evaluate and intervene with the workings of the complex sensory nervous system. For this reason, referrals to occupational therapists are common and absolutely warranted in many of these challenging cases. However, psychotherapists are specially trained to guide the cognitive-behavioral process and address the associated emotions of anxiety, depression, or fear. Furthermore, psychotherapists are uniquely qualified to complete a functional analysis of the presenting problems and develop a comprehensive treatment plan that targets the symptomatic behaviors, the dysfunction within the family system, and inappropriate reactions within the school environment. Psychotherapy provides a cohesive understanding of a child's nervous system and consequent emotions and behaviors, as well as a road map for making changes in problematic areas. Sometimes it is appropriate to refer a client to occupational therapy for a period of time before even starting therapy, while other times both can occur simultaneously. In other cases, the therapist is able to manage the sensory portion of the treatment without making a referral at all.

SUMMARY

This chapter has identified several red flags that may indicate the need to evaluate the sensory system and consider sensory dysregulation as a potential driving force for the targeted problematic behavior. In addition, common difficulties that may potentially arise in therapy have been discussed and troubleshooting strategies offered. It is important to remember that, as with all therapy interventions, each case is unique and each person arrives for therapy with a multitude of experiences, neurobiological hardwiring, genetic predispositions, cognitive beliefs, overt behaviors, and coping skills. As therapists it is our job to avoid making assumptions and consider each case as a unique investigation into the targeted behavior, its genesis, function, and reinforcing mechanisms. Considering sensory dysregulation as a potential factor can improve the success and depth of treatment in many of these complicated and challenging cases.

CHAPTER 10

Where Do We Go from Here?

This book has described the neurological phenomenon known as sensory dysregulation, where difficulties in the sensory nervous system impact psychological functioning resulting in a complicated therapeutic picture. A novel therapeutic approach has been described in detail that builds on empirically validated treatments to augment proven interventions so that they can positively impact these types of cases. Furthermore, numerous case studies were presented to illustrate the therapy process for different diagnostic presentations. Finally, common situations that interfere with therapy were discussed. This chapter reviews some of the ways sensory dysregulation can negatively impact a child's emotional and behavioral development, as well as positive aspects of this neurological phenomenon.

UNTREATED SENSORY DYSREGULATION

Left untreated, sensory dysregulation can cause lifelong struggles for individuals who don't understand how their nervous system is functioning and the problems it can cause.

Intimacy Problems

Interpersonal relationships can be negatively affected in people who experience sensory dysregulation. Anger, frustration, and extreme irritability interfere early in development with the establishment of relationships with both family and peers. Oppositional behavior, blaming others for internal discomfort, chronic irritability, and avoidance of environments that antagonize the nervous system can lead to isolation, feelings of low self-worth, and depression.

Those who seek out sensory stimuli may need to constantly be in the company of others, seek inappropriate sensory stimulation, or misunderstand social norms, leading to similar social and relationship dysfunction.

Family Discord

Having a child with a dysregulated nervous system can lead to family discord. Parents and siblings can feel unfairly burdened by the needs of the child. Parents may feel responsible for helping their child accomplish tasks that are inappropriate to the child's age and stage of development, such as putting socks on a teenager's feet, cutting up food, helping with bathing, or accompanying an older child to ask a question of a teacher or other adult. This can lead to anger and frustration that their child continues to require an excessive amount of parental attention, time, and energy despite the child's advanced age and stage of development. Siblings can feel embarrassed by the child's inappropriate behavior or burdened by demands placed on them (e.g., eating only at certain restaurants or having to always do the dishes for a sibling who cannot tolerate this task). Furthermore, conflicts erupt that can place blame on the child who is unable to tolerate his internal and/or external experience. Without accurate identification and appropriate treatment, effective problem-solving skills are not developed, conflicts and discord often disrupt family functioning, and behavioral and/or psychological disorders may worsen or persist for years.

EARLY INTERVENTION

Treating children with sensory challenges can give them a solid foundation for life. The therapeutic approach described in this book can provide children with lifelong skills that enable them to effectively manage their internal experiences and reactivity to sensory stimuli. Knowing how the body responds to stimuli by eliciting a fight, flight, or freeze response can help a child form a personalized understanding of her own nervous system and accept her unique sensory experience and functioning. Acceptance then leads to the creation of individualized, pleasant sensory experiences using a variety of sensory interventions. Soothing the nervous system allows one to approach previously challenging sensory experiences with an attitude of adventure and confidence. Understanding and accepting one's unique functioning allows for the moderation of sleep, activity level, eating, and lifestyle habits to support a healthy sensory system. Children who are able to learn and accept how their central nervous system operates and then create a lifestyle that uniquely meets their needs can often limit or completely eliminate the onset of co-occurring anxiety and the possible the development of behavioral disorders. Therapy helps these children and their families utilize their strengths to compensate for or diminish weaknesses, empowering children and leading to improved confidence.

Family functioning can also flourish as a result of therapeutic intervention. Challenging feelings and difficult behaviors are understood within the context of the sensory nervous system. Accommodating behaviors, negative reactions, or punishment of sensory-related behaviors can be eliminated. Furthermore, families learn to set appropriate boundaries and provide support, understanding, and encouragement to the sensory-sensitive child, leading to a more peaceful family environment. Healthy functioning also leads to enhanced relationships for the child throughout the lifespan. Children who manage their emotions and behaviors will grow up to be higher-functioning adults.

POSITIVE OUTCOMES
OF SENSORY DYSREGULATION

This book has described difficult-to-manage behaviors and emotions that often accompany the dysregulated nervous system. However, there are some important positive outcomes for children who have these quirky nervous systems. These characteristics should be

highlighted and celebrated in the context of therapy, and the therapist should inform the child and family about ways to utilize these
hardwired differences in productive and meaningful ways.

Empathy toward Others

Sensory dysregulation can lead to the development of compassion
and sensitivity toward others. Children with sensory dysregulation
may reach out when others are in need, knowing how uncomfortable, sad, and lonely it can be to go through a difficult time. When
their sensory issues are well regulated, these children are wonderful, supportive friends who are patient and accepting of individual
differences.

Artistic Ability

Having a sensitive nervous system can also contribute to great art-
istry. Children who are visually sensitive may have interesting and
unique ways of viewing a space or environment. These sensitivities
may enable them to demonstrate talent in visual arts such as interior design, graphic design, furniture design, computer graphics,
videography, performing arts, directing, photography, and archi-
tecture. Children who have sensitive auditory systems may be well
suited for a career in the music industry or, conversely, library science if noise is a problem. Reframing sensory dysregulation as a
possible pathway to a career can help the family adopt a more positive attitude toward the condition.

Creative Thinking

A sensitive nervous system may also contribute to an ability to
think creatively. Individuals with sensory sensitivities often possess
the ability to view a situation from multiple angles, think outside
the box, and solve problems creatively, talents that are useful in
a wide variety of professions and particularly helpful to entrepre-
neurs. Children who seek stimuli are better multitaskers and are
able to manage chaotic work environments in creative, productive
ways. Overall, these are highly talented and creative people whose

strengths should be nurtured and supported in order to help them realize their potential and become important contributors to society.

CONCLUSION

Misunderstood or misdiagnosed sensory dysregulation can be incredibly challenging to children, parents, and therapists. Although the occupational therapy world has long acknowledged the impact of the nervous system on a child's functioning, outside of the pervasive developmental disorders, psychology has overlooked this important piece of the therapy puzzle in terms of how these issues affect emotional and behavioral functioning. Consequently, children have been misunderstood and misdiagnosed, and treatment has been misguided in the therapy office. When treatment is unsuccessful, therapists can experience frustration, confusion, or feelings of helplessness that parallel the experience of the child and his family. The systematic evaluation, identification, and comprehensive treatment described in this book may make the difference between treatment failure and success. Early intervention helps families understand the nature of their children's behavior and teaches children how to master their nervous system. With these new skills, they can effectively manage their emotions and behaviors, utilize their strengths, and grow up to be productive, happy, adults.

References

Achenbach, T. M. (1991). *Manual for the Child Behavior Checklist/4–18 and 1991 Profile*. Burlington: Department of Psychiatry, University of Vermont

Ayres, A. J. (1958). The visual-motor function. *American Journal of Occupational Therapy, 12*, 130–138, 155.

Ayres, A. J. (1961). Development of the body scheme in children. *American Journal of Occupational Therapy, 15*, 99–102, 128.

Ayres, A. J. (1966a). Interrelation of perception, function, and treatment. *Journal of the American Physical Therapy Association, 46*, 741–744.

Ayres, A. J. (1966b). Interrelations among perceptual-motor abilities in a group of normal children. *American Journal of Occupational Therapy, 20*, 288–292.

Ayres, A. J. (1972a). Overview. In A. J. Ayres (Ed.), *Sensory integration and learning disorders* (pp. 1–12). Los Angeles: Western Psychological Services.

Ayres, A. J. (1972b). Some general principles of brain function. In A. J. Ayres (Ed.), *Sensory integration and learning disorders* (pp. 13–24). Los Angeles: Western Psychological Services.

Belluscio, B. A., Jin, L., Watters, V., Lee, T. H., & Hallett, M. (2011). Sensory sensitivity to external stimuli in Tourette syndrome patients. *Movement Disorders, 26*(14), 2538–2543.

Calkins, S. D., Fox, N. A., & Marshall, T. (1996). Behavioral and physiological antecedents of inhibited and diminished behavior. *Child Development, 67*, 523–540.

Davies, P. L., Chang, W. P., & Gavin, W. J. (2009). Maturation of sensory gating performance in children with and without sensory processing disorders. *International Journal of Psychophysiology, 72*(2), 187–197.

Davies, P. L., & Gavin, W. J. (2007). Validating the diagnosis of sensory processing disorders using EEG technology. *American Journal of Occupational Therapy, 61,* 176–189.

Dunn, W. (1999a). *The Sensory Profile.* San Antonio, TX: Pearson.

Dunn, W. (1999b). *Short Sensory Profile.* San Antonio, TX: Psychological Corporation.

Dunn, W. (2002). *Adolescent/Adult Sensory Profile.* San Antonio, TX: Therapy Skill Builders.

Dunn, W., & Daniels, D. B. (2002). Initial development of the infant/toddler sensory profile. *Journal of Early Intervention, 25*(1), 27–41.

Eddy, C. M., Rickards, H. E., Critchley, H. D., & Cavanna, A. E. (2013). A controlled study of personality and affect in Tourette syndrome. *Comprehensive Psychiatry, 54*(2), 105–110.

Fox, N. A., Henderson, H. A., Rubin, K. H., Calkins, S. D., & Schmidt, L. A. (2001). Continuity and discontinuity of behavioral inhibition and exuberance: Psychophysiological and behavioral influences across the first four years of life. *Child Development, 72,* 1–21.

Frassinetti, F., Bolognini, N., & Làdavas, E. (2002). Enhancement of visual perception by crossmodal visuo-auditory interaction. *Experimental Brain Research, 147,* 332–343.

Hopkins, J., Gouze, K. R., Sadhwani, A., Radtke, L., Labailly, S. A., & Lavigne, J. V. (2008, May). *Biological and psychosocial risk factors differentially predict internalizing/externalizing problems in preschoolers.* Paper presented at the 20th annual convention of the Association for Psychological Science, Chicago.

Kim, R. S., Seitz, A. R., & Shams, L. (2008). Benefits of stimulus congruency for multisensory facilitation of visual learning. *PLoS ONE, 3*(1), e1532.

Kisley, M. A., & Cornwell, Z. M. (2006). Gamma and beta neural activity evoked during a sensory gating paradigm: Effects of auditory, somatosensory and cross-modal stimulation. *Clinical Neurophysiology, 117*(11), 2549–2563.

Kranowitz, C. S. (2005). *The out-of-sync child: Recognizing and coping with sensory processing disorder.* New York: Skylight Press/Perigee.

Mansueto, C. S., & Keuler, D. J. (2005). Tic or compulsion?: It's Tourettic OCD. *Behavior Modification, 29*(5), 784–799.

McIntosh, D. N., Miller, L. J., Shyu, V., & Hagerman, R. (1999). Sensory-modulation disruption, electrodermal responses, and functional behaviors. *Developmental Medicine and Child Neurology, 41*, 608–615.

Meunier, S. A., & Tolin, D. F. (2009). The treatment of disgust. In B. O. Olatunji & D. McKay (Eds.), *Disgust and its disorders: Theory, assessment, and treatment implications* (pp. 271–284). Washington, DC: American Psychological Association.

Miller, L. J., Nielsen, D. M., Schoen, S. A., & Brett-Green, B. A. (2009). Perspectives on sensory processing disorder: A call for translational research. *Frontiers in Integrative Neuroscience, 3*, 22.

Miller, L. J., Reisman, J. E., McIntosh, D. N., & Simon, J. (2001). An ecological model of sensory modulation: Performance of children with fragile X syndrome, autistic disorder, attention-deficit/hyperactivity disorder, and sensory modulation dysfunction. In S. S. Roley, E. I. Blanche, & R. C. Schaaf (Eds.), *Understanding the nature of sensory integration with diverse populations* (pp. 57–88). San Antonio, TX: Therapy Skill Builders.

Miller, L. J., Robinson, J., & Moulton, D. (2004). Sensory modulation dysfunction: Identification in early childhood. In R. DelCarmen-Wiggins & A. Carter (Eds.), *Handbook of infant, toddler, and preschool mental health assessment* (pp. 247–270). New York: Oxford University Press.

Olatunji, B. O., Tart, C. D., Ciesielski, B. G., McGrath, P. B., & Smits, J. A. (2011). Specificity of disgust vulnerability in the distinction and treatment of OCD. *Journal of Psychiatric Research, 45*(9), 1236–1242.

Ozdemir, L., & Akdemir, N. (2009). Effects of multisensory stimulation on cognition, depression and anxiety levels of mildly-affected Alzheimer's patients. *Journal of the Neurological Sciences, 283*, 211–213.

Schneider, M. L., Moore, C. F., Gajewski, L. L., Laughlin, N. K., Larson, J. A., Gay, C. L., et al. (2007). Sensory processing disorders in a nonhuman primate model: Evidence of occupational therapy practice. *American Journal of Occupational Therapy, 61*, 247–253.

Stein, B. E., Huneycutt, W. S., & Meredith, M. A. (1988). Neurons and behavior: The same rules of multisensory integration apply. *Brain Research, 448*, 355–358.

Stein B. E., & Meredith M. A. (1993). *The merging of the senses.* Cambridge, MA: MIT Press.

Taylor, S., Conelea, C. A., McKay, D., Crowe, K. B., & Abramowitz, J. S. (2014). Sensory intolerance: Latent structure and psychopathologic correlates. *Comprehensive Psychiatry, 55*(5), 1279–1284.

Woods, D. W., Miltenberger, R. G., & Flach, A. D. (1996). Habits, tics, and stuttering: Prevalence and relation to anxiety and somatic awareness. *Behavior Modification, 20*(2), 216–225.

Wu, M. S., Lewin, A. B., Murphy, T. K., & Storch, E. A. (2014). Misophonia: Incidence, phenomenology, and clinical correlates in an undergraduate student sample. *Journal of Clinical Psychology, 70*(10), 994–1007.

Index

Page numbers followed by *f* indicate figure

Eye contact intervention, 83–85

F

Families
  impact of early intervention on,
    159
  multiple children having sensory
    dysregulation with different
    needs, 151
  untreated sensory dysregulation
    and family discord, 158
  See also Parents
Far senses
  dysregulation of, 23–27
  overview, 18–19
  specific interventions for over-
    and underresponsive children
    auditory, 85–86
    olfactory, 77–79
    tactile, 80–82
    taste sense, 79–80
    visual, 82–85
  See also specific senses
Food presentations, 79–80

G

Gag response interventions, 80
Games
  in counterconditioning, 72–73
  Where's Waldo? for visual
    dysregulation, 82
Generalized anxiety disorder
  (GAD)
  sensory dysregulation can mimic,
    41
  treatment specific to sensory
    dysregulation, 116–119
Guilt, 106

H

Habituation, 21
Hair brushing intervention, 81
Homeostasis, 3
Home spa experience, 81
House of horrors activity, 81
Human development, sensory
  dysregulation and, 14

I

Infant/Toddler Sensory Profile, 33
Information modulation, 20–22
Inhibition, 20
Intake evaluation, 31–33
Internal regulation assessment, 36*f*
Internal senses. *See* Near senses
Interoceptive sense
  description of, 19
  sensory dysregulation, 27
  specific interventions for over-
    and underresponsive children,
    86–87
Interpersonal and intimacy
  problems, 157–158

J

"Just right" obsessive–compulsive
  disorder, 47–48

L

Learning, importance of sensory
  regulation to, 4–5

M

Maladaptive behaviors
  parental accommodation of, 91–
    95
  parent–child interactions that
    reinforce, 149
  understanding the functional value
    of, 37–40
Messy rooms, 85
Misphonia, 56
Multiple diagnoses, 148
Multisensory integration, 3–4

N

Near senses
  dysregulation of, 27–29
  overview, 19
  specific interventions for over- and
    underresponsive children, 86–88
  See also Interoceptive sense;
    Proprioceptive sense; Vestibular
    sense